D0603804

CALGARY PUBLIC LIBRARY

JUL - - 2013

# vintage
## beauty parlor

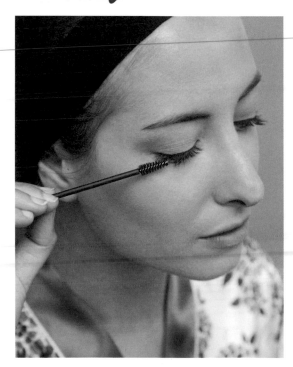

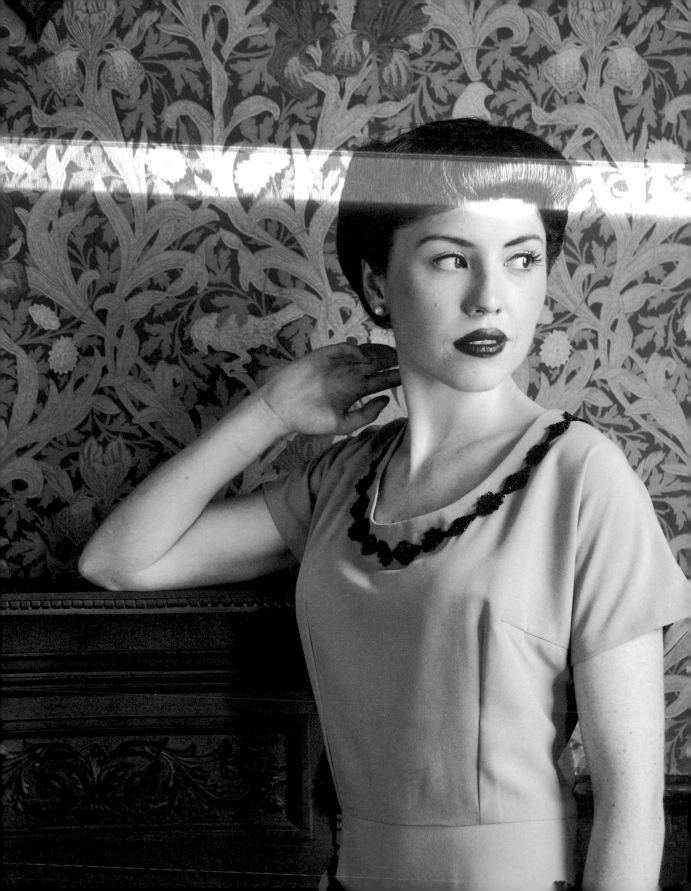

# vintage
## beauty parlor

**Flawless hair &
make-up in iconic
vintage styles**

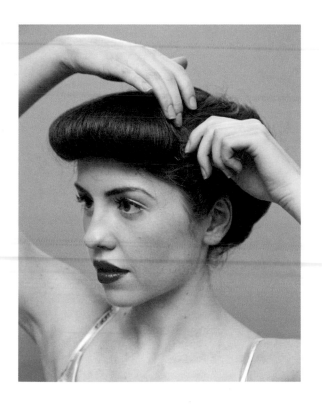

**Hannah Wing**
Photography by Penny Wincer

LONDON · NEW YORK

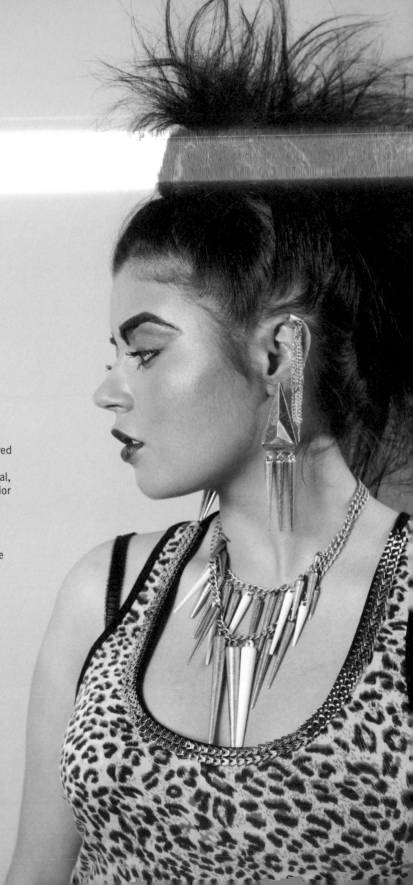

**Senior Designer** Sonya Nathoo
**Editor** Ellen Parnavelas
**Production** Gary Hayes
**Editorial Director** Julia Charles
Art Director Leslie Harrington

Make-up Artist and Stylist Liz Martins
**Hair Stylist** Katie Kendrick
**Indexer** Hilary Bird

First published in the UK in 2013
by Ryland Peters & Small
20–21 Jockey's Fields
London WC1R 4BW
and
519 Broadway, 5th Floor
New York, NY 10012
www.rylandpeters.com
10 9 8 7 6 5 4 3 2 1

Text copyright © Hannah Wing 2013
Design and photographs copyright
© Ryland Peters & Small 2013

The author's moral rights have
been asserted. All rights reserved. No part
of this publication may be reproduced, stored
in a retrieval system, or transmitted in any
form or by any means, electronic, mechanical,
photocopying, or otherwise, without the prior
permission of the publisher.

ISBN: 978–1-84975–362–3

A CIP record for this book is available from the
British Library.

Library of Congress Cataloging-in-Publication
Data has been applied for.

Printed in China.

# Contents

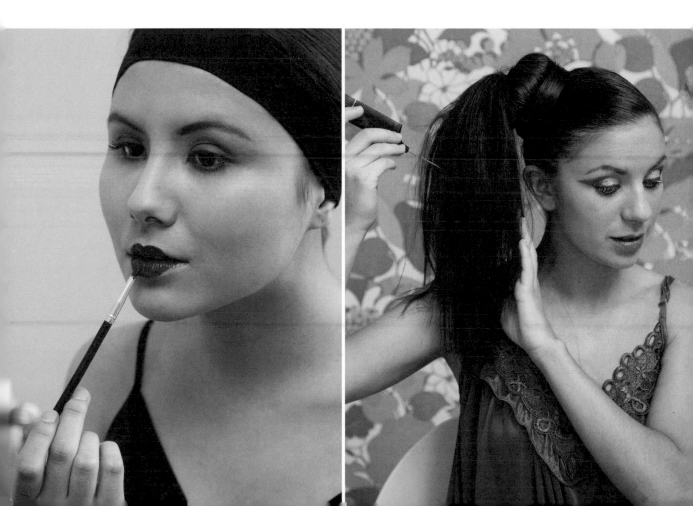

# Beauty Through the Decades

Perfect pouts, bedroom eyes, glowing skin and lustrous hair – oh how we long to be as glamorous as screen sirens such as Marilyn Monroe and Grace Kelly. I have no doubt that my childhood obsession with classic films shaped my interest in the world of fashion and beauty as I recall spending hours studying the immaculate style of stars such as Elizabeth Taylor, Lauren Bacall, Audrey Hepburn and Sophia Loren.

I am certainly not the only one who has sought to emulate the inspiring fashion and beauty styles presented to us from the big screens of days gone by – especially in recent years. Vintage styles from throughout the twentieth century have become highly fashionable, with victory rolls and finger waves, beehives and backcombing making a comeback on the high street as well as the catwalk. With celebrities such as Lana Del Ray, Adele and Paloma Faith championing classic fashion and beauty styles, all things vintage have become far less of an idiosyncrasy and much more a part of mainstream culture.

Embracing nostalgia is not a new phenomenon, however. It was during the late 1970s that people first began to tire of modern mass-produced fashion, as well as realizing the financial benefits of recycling. Trawling through thrift stores to seek out high-quality style statements suddenly became acceptable. Flea markets and jumble sales became prevalent and shopping for pre-worn items was no longer considered a misfortune of the poor, but a skilled pastime for those with a well-trained eye.

Quick-thinking fashion designers seized this opportunity to release collections inspired by designs seen in the 1940s, which were gratefully received by those who did not relish spending hours sifting through rails of second-hand clothes with the faint scent of moth balls. Others saw a business opportunity and it wasn't long before garments were being traded in specialist vintage outlets for large sums of money, based on the exclusivity of the pieces. Stylists, individuals and celebrities were regularly seen searching for vintage couture treasures at trendy locations such as Portobello Road in London and Les Puces de Saint-Ouen in Paris, something which has remained unchanged to this day.

Electing to re-create a look from a bygone era need not require the retrogression of your entire wardrobe, hair and make-up kit, but can be easily achieved with tools that are widely available today, using simple techniques that can be mastered with a bit of knowledge and guidance. Admittedly, achieving a glamorous look from yesteryear may involve beauty and hairstyling techniques that demand a little more time to perfect, but I feel that the reward far outweighs the commitment.

The following pages will explore the hair and make-up styles of each decade from the 1920s to the 1980s, with background information about the fashion and beauty of each period, alongside specific hair and make-up looks that can be re-created at home following the step-by-step instructions. In addition, you will find tips on clothing, accessories, shoes and even fragrance, as well as a list of suppliers of original and reproduction vintage items to assist you in achieving your chosen look, making it easy for you to become a vintage style icon in no time.

Before you get started, you can use the timeline overleaf as a quick reference guide to fashion designers and specific trends in each decade. I recommend that you experiment with looks from different eras, as you will find that your hair length, face shape and figure will dictate what works best for you. I sincerely hope you enjoy re-creating the looks as much as I did.

Hannah Wing

# Timeline of Key Trends

*Discover your favourite vintage looks using this quick reference timeline to help you identify the key trends and fashion designers in each decade.*

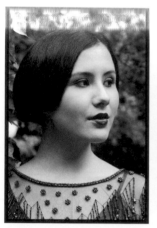 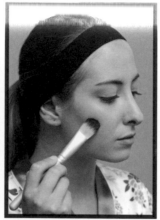 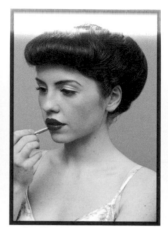 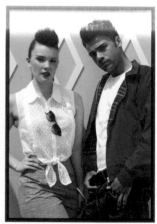

## 1920s

*'Comme de garçon'* and 'flapper' style were the trends followed by the young and the beautiful throughout the decade. Designers Jean Lanvin, Salvatore Ferragamo and Jean Patou competed fiercely to achieve the most desirable couture, while Coco Chanel made a name for herself with wardrobe staples such as the little black dress and the twinset.

## 1930s

Hollywood movie-star glamour dominated the thirties, with names like Elsa Schiaparelli, Madeleine Vionnet and Cristóbal Balenciaga commanding the fashion stage. Schiaparelli adopted many of her ideas from Surrealism, with sketches by Salvador Dalí and Jean Cocteau printed or embroidered on her dresses.

## 1940s

Wartime necessitated practical clothing, so an understated but feminine look prevailed in the earlier part of the decade. Rationed fashion was created by designers such as Edward Molyneux, Hardy Amies and Norman Hartnell. In contrast, the delicate and feminine post-war 'New Look' was created by Christian Dior as the forties drew to a close.

## 1950s

Mainstream fashion trends placed an emphasis on femininity with designers such as Pierre Balman and Jacques Fath in great demand. Later in the decade, rock 'n' roll grew in popularity among the youth, and 'rockers' and 'beatniks' stirred up a storm as the diversity in subcultures began to expand.

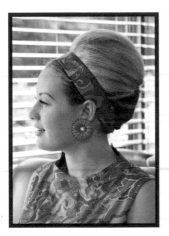

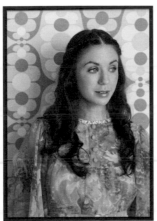

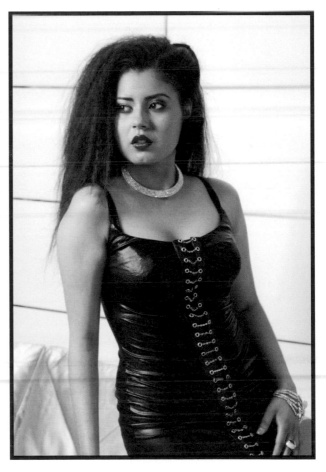

## 1960s

During the sixties, subcultures were popping up all over the place and 'hippies', 'mods' and 'northern soulers' provided a range of fashion options. Designer Mary Quant famously raised the hems of skirts and dresses to shocking heights. Other notable sixties designers include André Courréges, Barbara Hulanicki and Emilio Pucci.

## 1970s

The seventies saw the aggression of Punk, the simplicity of ethnic-inspired looks, the glitter of disco and the androgyny of Glam Rock, creating a myriad of fashion styles for individuals to experiment with. Kenzo Takada, Sonia Rykiel and Hubert de Givenchy were some of the decade's most notable designers.

## 1980s

New Romantic and 'gothic' were the dominant subcultures of the 1980s. Versace, Ralph Lauren and Calvin Klein were the decade's prominent designers.

# Basic Hair and Make-up Techniques
## application of base

*Base make-up will give your skin an even tone, covering any blemishes or dark circles.*

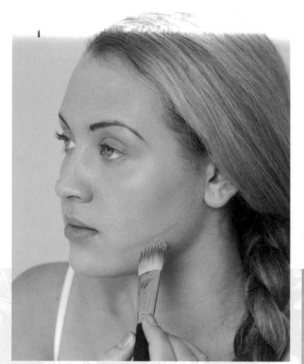

1 Using your fingertips, apply a face primer all over your face, working it into the skin to reduce fine pores. A dry prepare your skin for the application of foundation, as well as helping your make-up last longer. Colour match your foundation along your jawline using a foundation brush.

2 Apply concealer using your fingertip or a concealer brush to mask any blemishes or dark circles. I like to keep a yellow, green and mauve concealer wheel in my make-up kit as different colour concealers will even the skin tone in different ways: yellow lightens dark circles, green balances excessive redness and mauve has a skin-brightening effect.

3 Apply foundation evenly all over your face with a foundation brush. Use the flat edge of the brush in sweeping motions to ensure an even blend of colour.

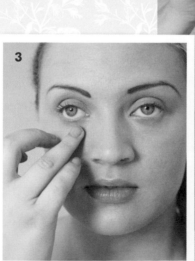

# blusher and bronzer

*Blusher can be applied on different parts of your cheeks, but always keep the colour in an area where you would naturally flush. Bronzer should only be applied to areas that would naturally catch the sun, such as your cheeks, forehead, bridge of your nose and chin — not the whole face.*

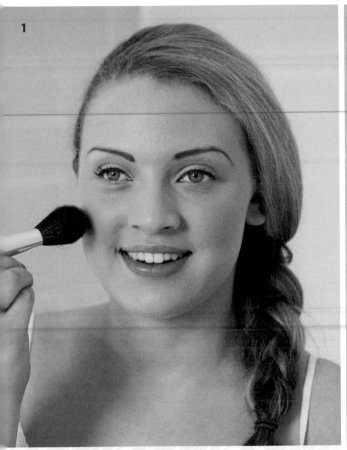

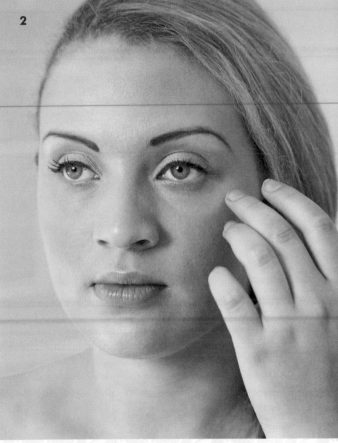

**1** Sweep a large, domed brush over your powder blusher or bronzer. Tap the brush before applying to remove any excess powder from the bristles. Smile so that the 'apples' of your cheeks are prominent and apply blusher or bronzer directly to that area, blending with circular motions.

**2** If you are using a crème blusher or bronzer, use the pads of your index and middle fingers to blend the colour evenly.

**3** Finish by applying a light dusting of translucent powder over your face with a large domed brush to set.

# basic eye make-up

*Before applying any eye make-up, gently pat on an eye primer, being careful not to drag the delicate skin. This will create an even surface for your eye make-up.*

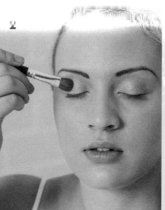 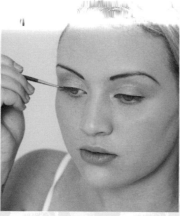 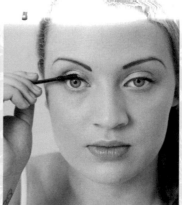 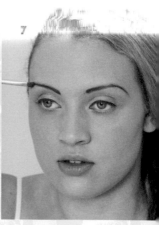

**1** Using a concealer or foundation brush, apply concealer and foundation to the whole eye area all the way up to the brow bone. This will create an even skin tone. Apply a light dusting of translucent powder using a small domed brush to set your base before applying your eye-shadow.

**2** Apply eye-shadow in a colour of your choice over the whole eye socket using a flat, round-edged eye-shadow brush. Apply a second colour, as desired to emphasize the outer corner of the eye or to add depth to the socket crease.

**3** If you are using false lashes, apply them with tweezers according to the manufacturer's instructions at this point.

**4** Apply eyeliner to your eyelids, as close to the upper lash line as possible. Use a liquid or gel eyeliner if you are using false lashes, or a kohl pencil eyeliner for a softer, more natural look.

**5** Apply mascara to your lashes, ensuring that you lift the lashes from the root. Apply a second coat, if desired. Mascara isn't always necessary if you are wearing false

lashes – simply use a lash comb to blend your natural lashes in with the false ones.

**6** Apply eyeliner to your lower lash line at this point, if you wish. For a soft, long-lasting smoky effect, use a small, square-tipped brush to line your lower lash line with black or brown eye-shadow. Gently pull the lower lash line downwards to line the rim with a soft kohl liner.

**7** Tidy your brows using a brow comb, then use a small, angled brush to define them with brown or black brow powder or eye-shadow. Gently comb your brows again and set with translucent powder or clear mascara.

**8** Use a soft brush to remove any excess eye-shadow from around the eye area.

# applying lipstick and gloss

*A good lip liner will help your lipstick last longer and prevent it from 'bleeding', enabling you to shape your lips to make them fuller or slimmer, depending on your preference. Choose a lip liner in a shade as close to your lipstick as possible. Sharpen your lip liner and blunt the tip on the back of your hand before using.*

**1** Outline your lips with the lip liner, applying it to the edge of the natural lip line to make your lips look smaller or the outer edge of the natural lip line to make your lips look bigger. Correct any imperfections to the natural lip line as you go and concentrate on making the shape symmetrical, especially the cupid's bow. When you are happy with the shape, fill your lips entirely with liner to make your lip colour last longer.

**2** Apply an even coat of lipstick in your chosen shade using a lip brush for greater precision. Blot your lips with a tissue, then apply a second coat of lipstick. Blot your lips again to seal in the colour.

**3** Apply clear lip gloss to the centre of the lips, as desired, to make your lips shine and create an illusion of fullness. However, omit this step you would like to maintain a more matte effect.

*Lip gloss catches the light and makes the lips appear fuller.*

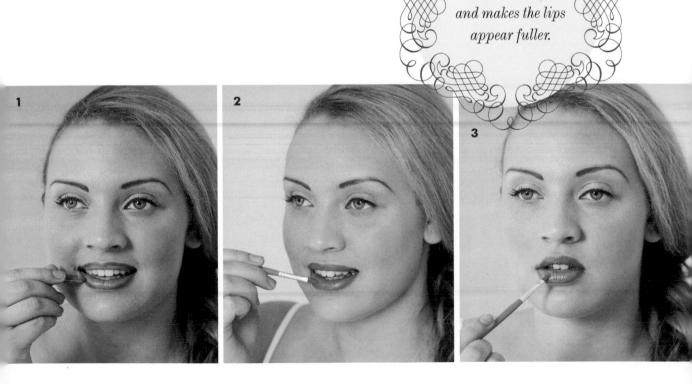

# three ways to create curls

*Whether you want sexy, voluminous curls, soft beachy waves or neat, vintage-style rolls, there are many different ways to curl your hair and each one will yield different results. Try each of these methods to see which works best for your hair.*

### USING ROLLERS

The position in which you place your rollers will determine the overall appearance of your finished hairstyle. To create maximum volume, for example, it is essential that the rollers are set directly over the roots of your hair.

The direction in which you roll the hair will also affect the result; putting in your rollers working from the parting at the top of your head down both sides will create root lift

and add volume to the width of your style, whereas putting in your rollers moving from the top of your head towards the back will create root lift and add depth. Use different-sized rollers to create tighter or looser curls – the smaller the roller, the tighter the curl.

Always allow your rollers to cool down fully before removing them, as this will set the curls, creating a longer-lasting finish and preventing the curls from dropping.

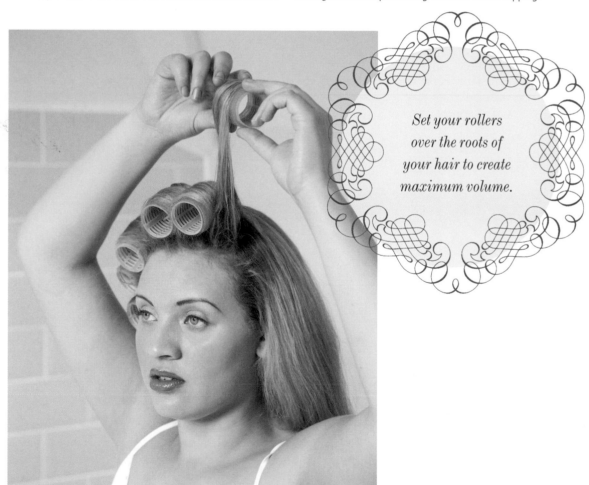

*Set your rollers over the roots of your hair to create maximum volume.*

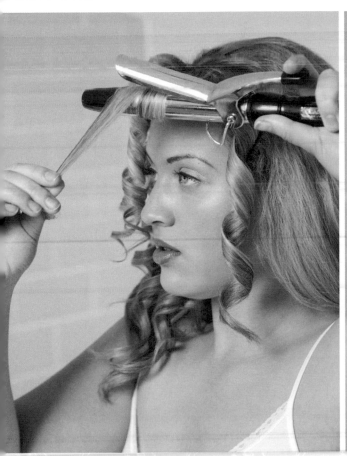

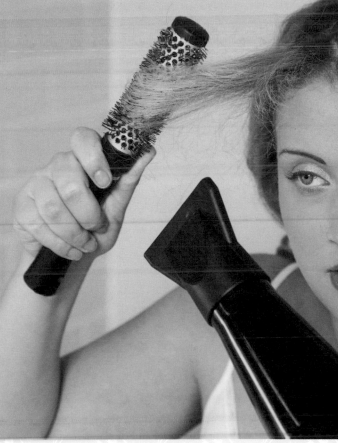

## USING A CURLING IRON

Not everyone has time to pin curl or roll their hair and wait for it to set, so using a curling iron is the perfect time-saving solution to create long-lasting curls in minutes.

Use different-sized curling irons to create tighter or looser curls – the smaller the iron, the tighter the curl.

Take a small section of hair and twist it around the iron. For long hair, wrap the hair around the iron from roots to tips. For short hair, wrap the hair from tips to roots. Hold your hair in the curling iron for 10-15 seconds before releasing it. Repeat with the rest of your hair.

## USING A ROUND BRUSH AND HAIRDRYER

Divide your hair into small sections to make styling easier. Choose the size of your round brush based on your hair length and the size of curl you wish to achieve. The tighter the curl, the smaller the brush you should use.

Brush each section of hair from roots to tips and roll the hair under and around the brush while blow-drying with hot air. Blow-dry the hair with it wrapped around the brush until it is completely dry, then blast with cold air. Hair should be dry and cool before removing the brush. Repeat with the rest of your hair.

## using a hair donut

*A hair donut is a great tool for creating the height and volume required for a variety of vintage hairstyles, such as beehives and other sixties-style 'updos'.*

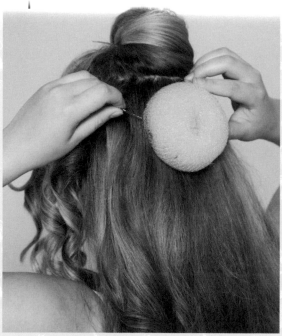 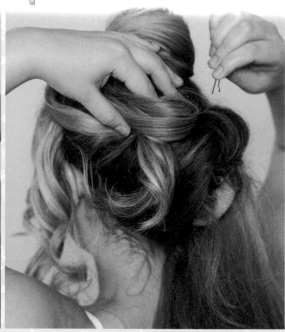

**1** Using a hair donut in this way is best suited to mid-length and longer hair.

To create an illusion of fullness and volume, place the donut on the area of your head you wish your hair to be raised. Insert hair grips/bobby pins all the way around the donut, to ensure that it is held securely in position.

**2** Gently backcomb the section of your hair that you will use to cover the donut from the roots to mid-way along its length. Using a soft-bristled hairbrush, lightly sweep the backcombed hair over the dougnut so it is completely covered. Pin your hair into the donut in the style of your choice, making sure that the donut is hidden from view.

# creating victory rolls

*Named after the fighter-plane manoeuvre of World War II, the victory-roll hairstyles of the forties and fifties always look elegant. Don't be put off by the fact that they look complicated – they are actually quite easy, once you know how.*

**1** Section off the hair that you want to use to create the roll and clip the rest of your hair out of the way.

To make it easier to roll the hair, curl the hair in the direction you want to roll it using a curling iron. Gently tease the curled hair into shape with a fine-tooth comb.

Insert a line of hair grips/bobby pins at the roots of the section where you wish to place your roll. Roll the section upwards, around your fingers.

**2** Pin the roll in place, securing the hair with hair grips/bobby pins on the inside of the roll. This will hold the roll and ensure that the hair grips/bobby pins are not visible.

Spray the roll with plenty of hairspray, then smooth away any stray hairs using a hairbrush to create a neat and tidy finish. Repeat this process if you would like to create more than one victory roll.

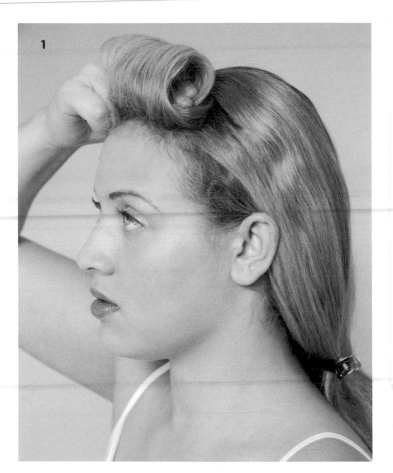

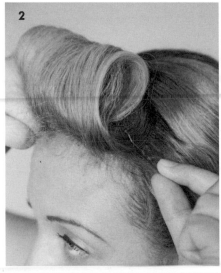

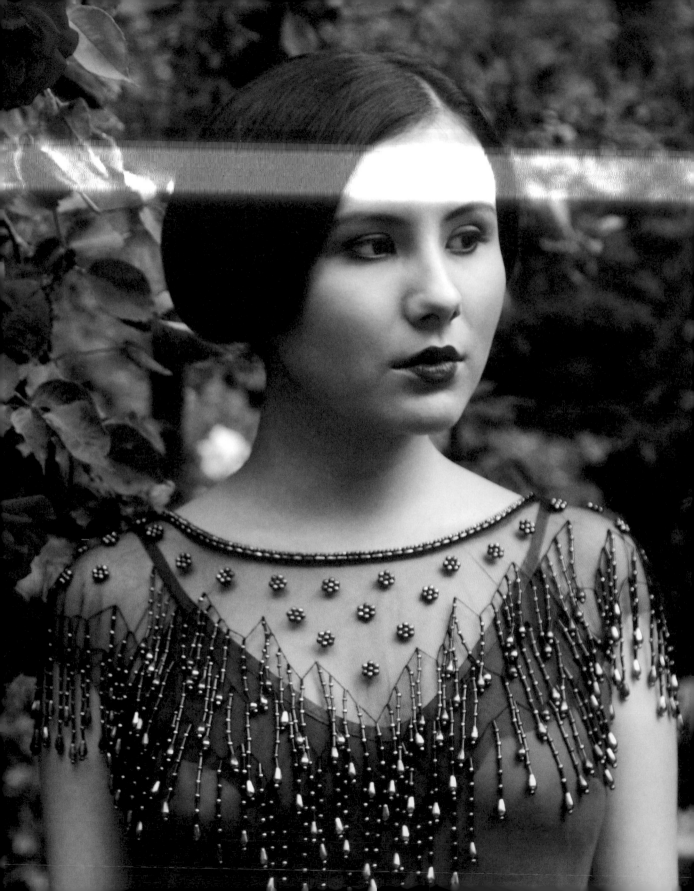

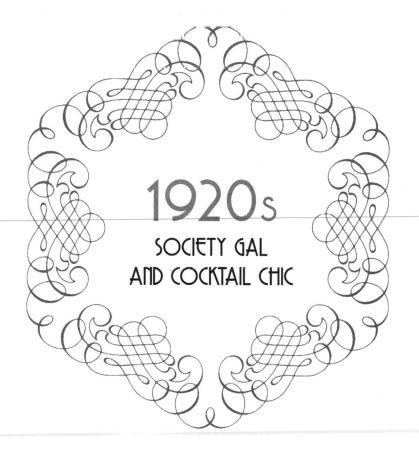

# 1920s
## SOCIETY GAL
## AND COCKTAIL CHIC

*The fusion of heavy tobacco and sweet-smelling*
*perfume conjure the aroma of the 'roaring twenties'.*
*Known as the 'Jazz Age', the 1920s was a time filled with*
*frivolity, music, dancing, cocktails, underground parties,*
*sumptuous colours and ground-breaking changes for*
*women — especially in fashion and beauty.*

# THE ROARING TWENTIES

It was during the 1920s that the longstanding prudish values of the Victorian era took shelter and as women were reminded that to secure a husband it was imperative that they created an alluring appearance. As a result, more dramatic make-up came into fashion so the emphasis of facial beauty changed from the natural and virginal to the enhanced and erotic.

Advances in cinema during the 1920s can also be held responsible for the increase in make-up sales. Until 1927, film was silent and made with limited light and camera technology, which served to mask the beauty of actresses. With the advancement of film during the 1920s, stars such as Marion Davies and Lillian Gish could be seen in all their glory. Actresses Clara Bow and Louise Brooks pushed the boundaries, wearing heavy cosmetics accompanied by ascending hemlines and hair length, and their then-controversial style whipped up an exciting storm. The columns of *Vanity Fair* and *Vogue* dedicated themselves to the details of the latest cutting-edge fashion and beauty, and set the foundations for media influence on the masses.

Long, flowing locks were cropped into sharp-edged plain bobs, which soon evolved into shingled bobs and pin-curled styles. As hairdressers got inventive, the demand for semi-permanent waving grew, although it remained a costly process only affordable to the rich.

Make-up, although less of a drain on the purse strings, was also quite indispensable to the modern look, albeit with less sophistication than it is today. Some women created artfully, although others used burned matchstick debris mixed with petroleum jelly as a means of darkening their lashes and crushed geranium or poppy petals to make cheek and lip tints.

Underneath the make-up, women aspired to a healthy, flawless complexion, so it was no surprise that skincare products were also marketed in abundance. During this period, women were coerced into trying cold cream cleansers, face masks and blotting papers in an attempt to achieve the porcelain-like skin that was fashionable at the time. Ivory-coloured powder was sometimes applied to the face to create the pale comeplexion that was desirable for twenties make-up styles.

By 1909, Helena Rubinstein had arrived in London, having already taken the beauty markets of Australia and Europe by storm. Her London emporium positioned her as an expert in the issues of 'problem' skin types, with her bestselling Crème Valaze and the mantra that 'there are no ugly women, just lazy ones'. Her products adorned the dressing tables of many a sophisticated debutante, until Elizabeth Arden and Charles Revson, the founder of Revlon, also began to command the skincare and cosmetics stage.

*make-up colour palette:*

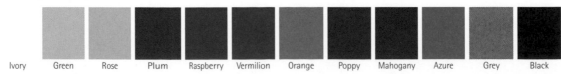

| Ivory | Green | Rose | Plum | Raspberry | Vermilion | Orange | Poppy | Mahogany | Azure | Grey | Black |

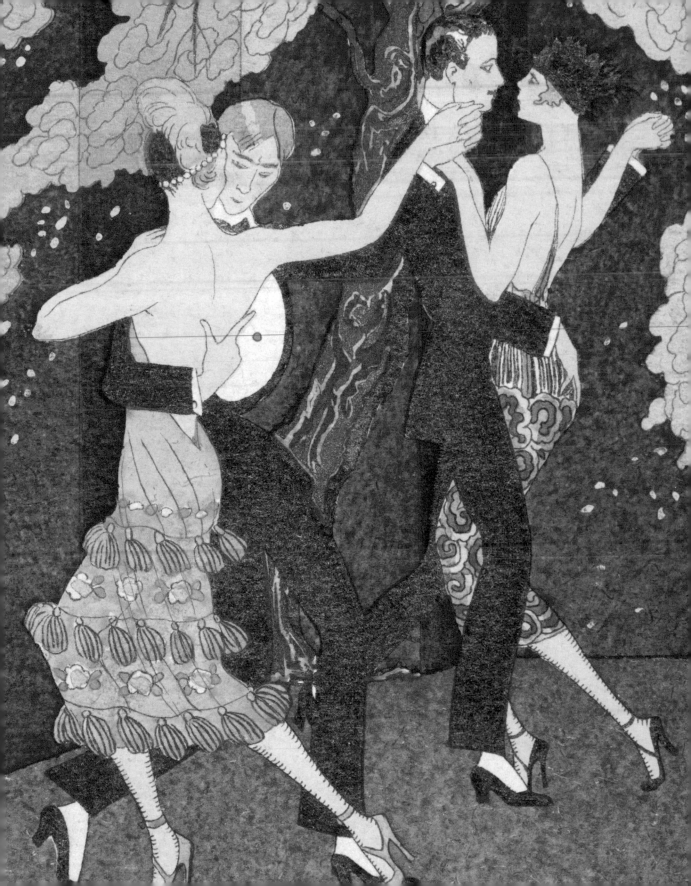

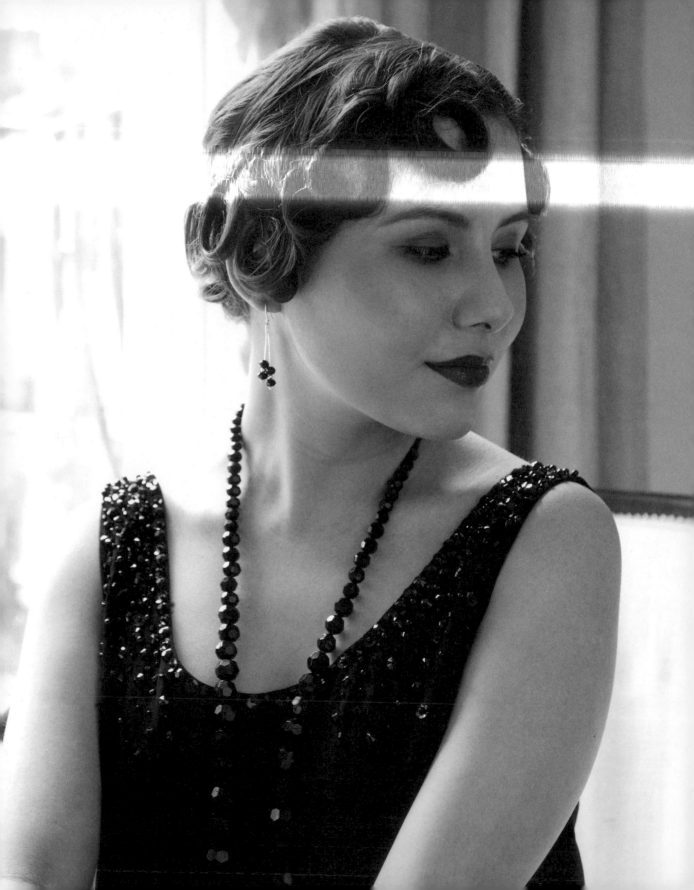

# SOCIETY GAL

*Soft-focus, monochrome pictures of beautiful starlets filled the high-society magazines that were poured over with excitement by women across the class barriers throughout the 1920s.*

This glamorous look reflects the confident, sultry yet coy image that women aspired to during this period. Perfect for a cocktail party or any smart evening occasion, a fun and elegant ensemble such as this will guarantee you are dressed to impress.

Intense eye make-up with smoky, kohl-lined eyes and sultry grey eye-shadow and strong, dark lips works well with the simplicity of this outfit – a little black dress, embellished with beads and feathers. Coco Chanel unwittingly championed sun-kissed skin in the latter part of the decade, but those with fairer complexions can carry this look with confidence, too as pale skin was fashionable throughout the twenties.

Ensure that your pin curls fall in part on your face as they will act as a frame for your features, which are guaranteed to look amazing under the warm glow of candlelight in the nearest jazz café.

## TO CREATE THIS LOOK YOU WILL NEED:

### MAKE UP
Large eye-shadow brush ✳ matte grey eye-shadow ✳ black kohl eyeliner pencil ✳ small, pointed eye-shadow brush or cotton bud/Q-tip ✳ black mascara ✳ lash and brow comb

### HAIR
Hairbrush ✳ pin curl clips ✳ curling iron ✳ pin-tail comb for sectioning ✳ hair grips/bobby pins ✳ hairspray

# SULTRY EYES

*Before applying your eye make-up, prepare your skin with a base coat*
*of foundation and concealer according to the directions on page 10. For an*
*authentic 1920s look, this should be matte to appear fresh and blemish free.*

1 Using a large cosmetic brush, apply a wash of grey eye-shadow over your eye socket. Work in circular motions to blend the eye-shadow upwards and outwards. Repeat this until you have your desired density of colour. Remember to apply each wash of colour lightly, as it is easier to build up colour than it is to remove it.

2 Sharpen a soft black eye pencil and test the point on the back of your hand. Use the pencil to apply eyeliner all around the eyes, outlining your upper and lower lash lines, working into the roots of the lashes to fill any gaps. Work from the inner corner of the eye outwards both underneath the eye and on the upper lash line.

**1**

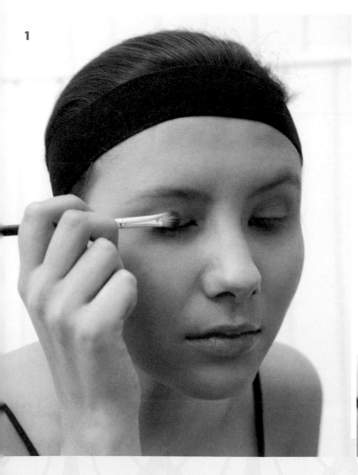

**2**

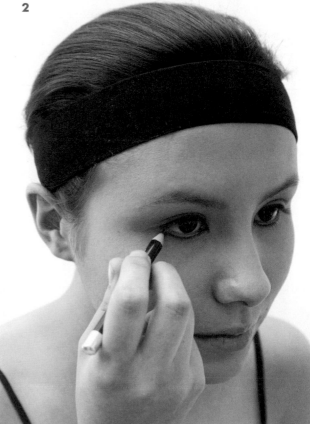

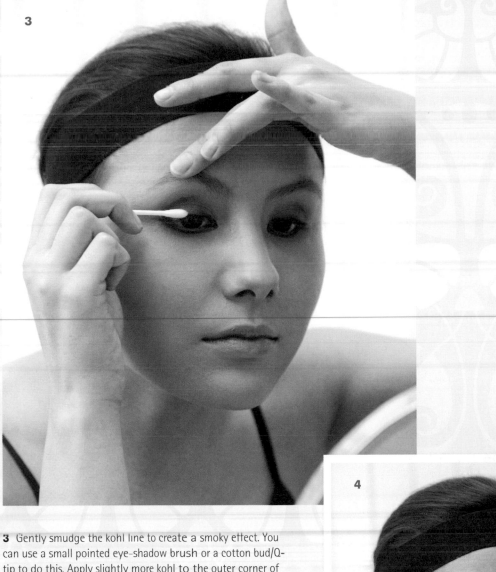

**3** Gently smudge the kohl line to create a smoky effect. You can use a small pointed eye-shadow brush or a cotton bud/Q-tip to do this. Apply slightly more kohl to the outer corner of the lash lines to increase the density of colour there.

**4** Apply a generous coat of black mascara to the lashes and allow to dry before applying the next coat. Once the lashes are dry, gently comb them through to remove any clumps. Apply another coat of mascara, allow it to dry and comb through the lashes again. Apply as many coats of mascara as desired, but for this look, you will need a minimum of two coats.

# PERFECT PIN CURLS

*For best results when curling your hair, leave it unwashed for at least a day*
*before styling and avoid using conditioner or it will be too soft to curl.*

1  Brush through the hair then, using the metal-pronged comb, take a horseshoe section of hair from the centre to the front of the head and pin it away to one side. Using a curling iron, curl the rest of the hair in small sections (see page 15). Make sure you curl the hair under with a slight root drag so that you don't create volume at the roots and the hair remains close to the head. Pin the individual curls into place as you go with pin curl clips.

2  Curl the front section of hair, as before, making sure to curl the hair under so the roots are flat, as before. Pin the individual curls into place and allow all the hair to cool and set. Make sure you are generous with the cooling time, as this will prolong the life of the curl.

3  Once the hair is, cool remove all the pins and section the hair off from the front to the back.

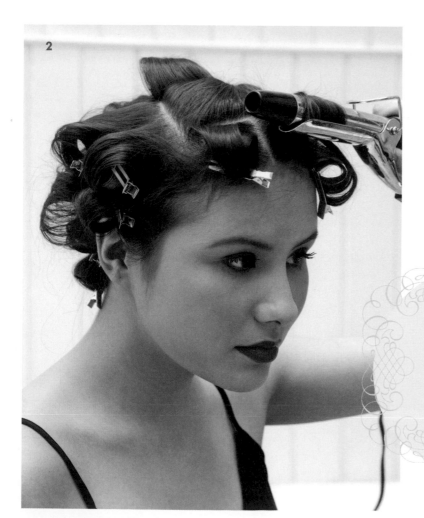

*Delicate curls pinned around the face act as a frame for your features.*

**4**

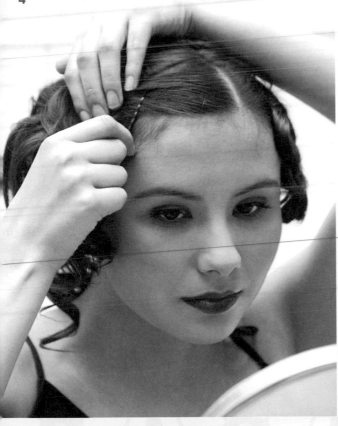

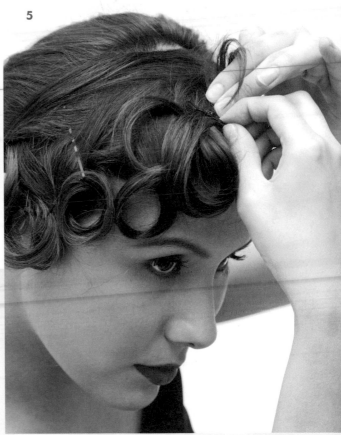

**5**

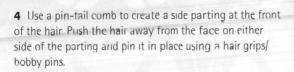

**4** Use a pin-tail comb to create a side parting at the front of the hair. Push the hair away from the face on either side of the parting and pin it in place using a hair grips/bobby pins.

**5** Spray each individual curl on either side of the parting with hairspray. Then bring the curls forward onto to forehead, creating a frame around the face. Secure the curls in place using hair grips/bobby pins. The curls should lay flat against the head, along the edges of the face

**6** Spray the individual curls at the back of the head with hairspray. Work around the rest of the head, pinning the individual curls into place all the way around the hairline. All the curls should be pinned flat against the head.

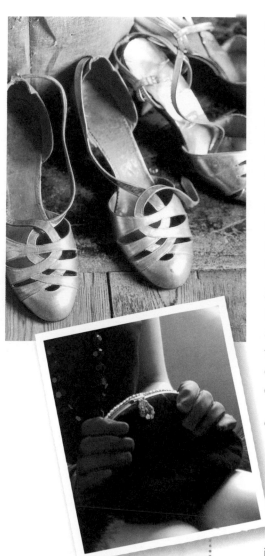

### occasion gloves

Elegant gloves, often in satin or lace, should be close fitting and can vary in finishing length from the wrist to the crook of the arm. To establish your glove size, take a tape measure and wrap it around your hand, just below your knuckles. Draw your hand into a fist shape and round up the measurement to the nearest number in inches. Naturally, some original vintage gloves don't have sizes and will often be made of non-stretch materials, so it is always helpful to try them on to check how comfortable they are.

### cocktail rings

Large and ornate in design, cocktail rings are statement pieces that were worn over gloves. Styles can vary, although Art Deco designs are the most fitting for an authentic 1920s look.

### bags

Complete any 1920s outfit with a small clutch bag. Snake and alligator skin were at the height of fashion, but it is important that you consider the practcalities of purchasing authentic antiques over faux reproductions. Tapestry bags or ornate velvet and beaded designs on long metal chains were equally popular.

### compacts

With the public application of make-up touch-ups being such a prominent trend in the1920s, any self-respecting society gal owned a compact. The style and design should be in keeping with the period, as compacts remained highly fashionable well into the 1960s. There is a large collectors' market for authentic pieces, so check antiques fairs and online auctions, but keep in mind that modern reproductions can be purchased for a fraction of the price.

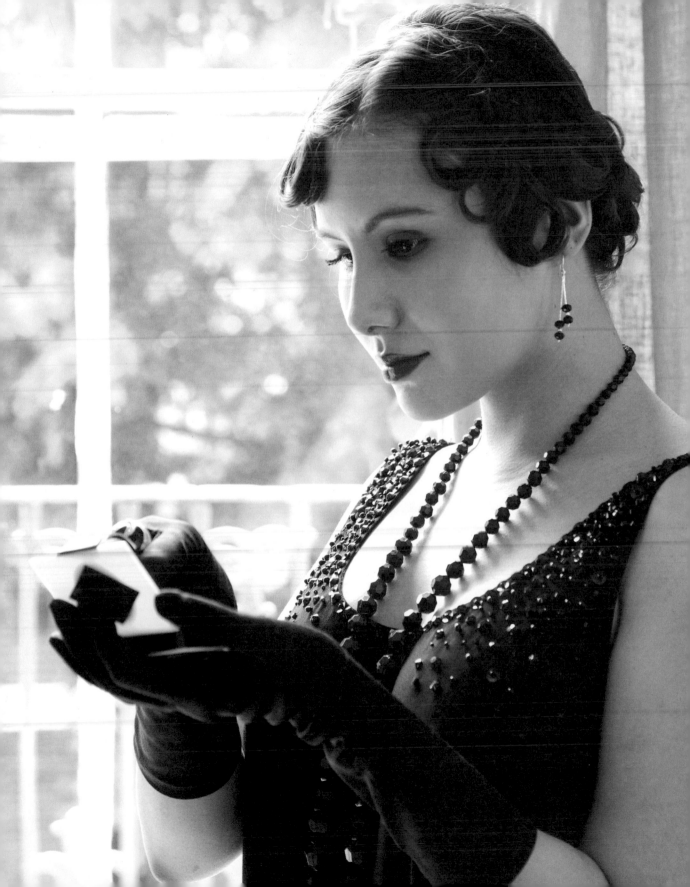

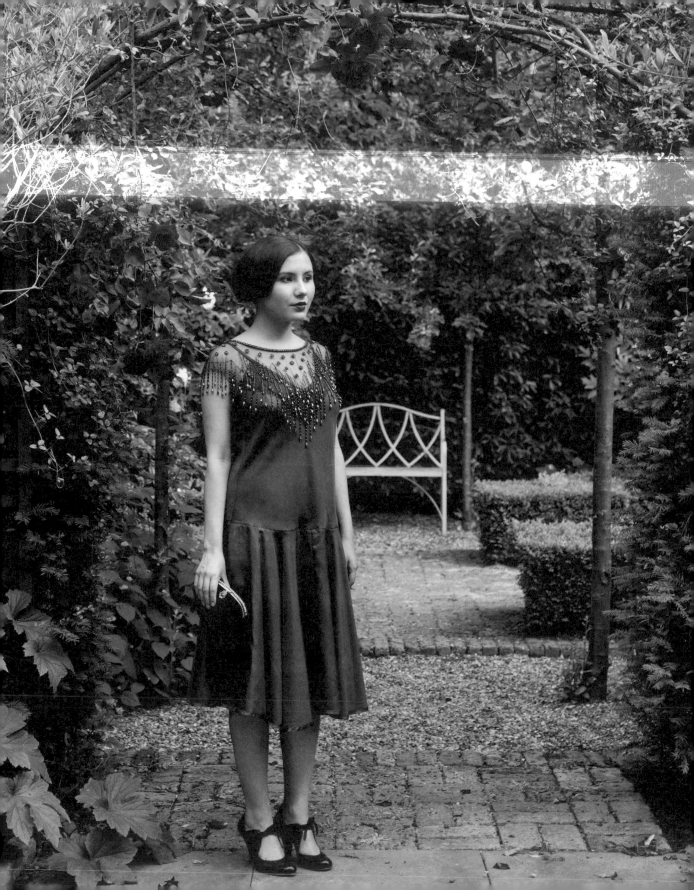

# COCKTAIL CHIC

*This elegant ensemble represents that typically seen around the middle of the decade, when radical changes to feminine fashion were presenting ladies with a newly acquired sense of self.*

A short, simple bob – or 'faux bob' for longer hair – together with pronounced make-up, creates the dramatic visual that dominated the decadent 1920s. The finished look is simply perfect for gathering with friends for dinner or early-evening cocktails around the gramophone.

Elfin hairstyles worn close to the head were the height of fashion during the decade, with many women chopping off their tresses in favour of a controversial bobbed haircut. The rebellious change in hair fashion in the 1920s signified the start of a major change in social norms and values – especially for women.

Block-colour eye-shadow, often in dark shades of grey or green, was worn with heavy kohl eyeliner and lashings of mascara build a strong frame around the eyes, while skin is matte and blemish-free. Place specific emphasis on creating a small, full lip, defined with a dark colour that accentuates the 'doll-like' pout favoured at the time.

## TO CREATE THIS LOOK YOU WILL NEED:

### MAKE-UP
Foundation * foundation brush * deep red or plum lip liner * dark red or plum matte lipstick * lip brush * tissues to blot * cleansing wipe or cotton bud/Q-tip

### HAIR
Heated rollers * hairbrush * fine-tooth comb * sectioning clips * hair grips/bobby pins * hairspray

# CUPID'S BOW LIPS

*For an authentic 1920s evening look, create the luscious illusion of Cupid's-bow lips in a deep shade of plum. Match them with the sultry eyes created on page 24. Try toning the matte grey eye-shadow with a deep mauve.*

1 Using a foundation brush, apply foundation to the entire lip area to mask the natural lip line. It is important that you stretch your lips to blend the foundation into the creases, as this will create an even surface as well as acting as a primer for the lip liner and lipstick.

2 Using a plum lip liner, mark out a point inside the width of your natural lip line. Draw the outline of the cupid's bow onto the lips, pronouncing the rise and fall of the centre of the top lip. Join the top and bottom lines so that your lips appear smaller.

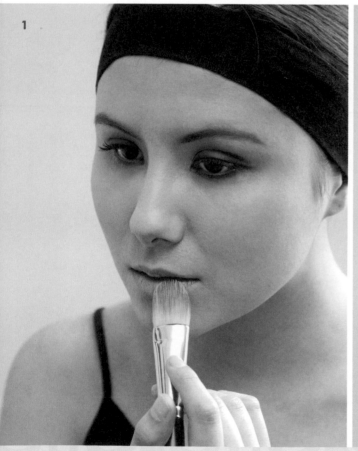

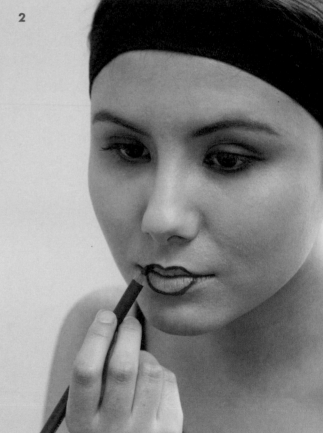

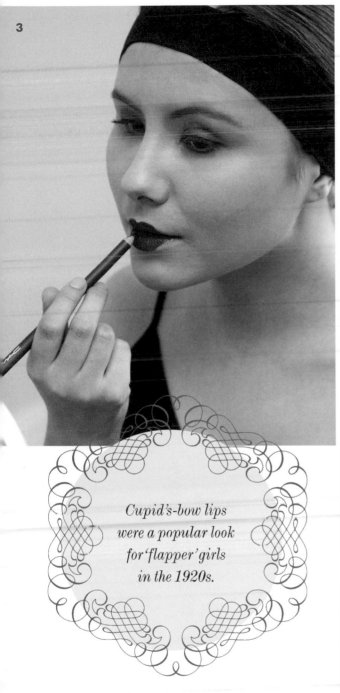

3

**3** Fill in the newly created cupid's-bow shape using the lip liner. If necessary, correct any mistakes by wrapping a cleansing wipe over a cotton bud/Q-tip and wiping them away. Make sure that both sides are exact mirror images of each other so that the shape is symmetrical.

**4** Apply a dark shade of red or plum matte lipstick with a lip brush for precision. Blot the lips with a tissue to remove any excess and apply a second coat of lipstick. Blot again to finish.

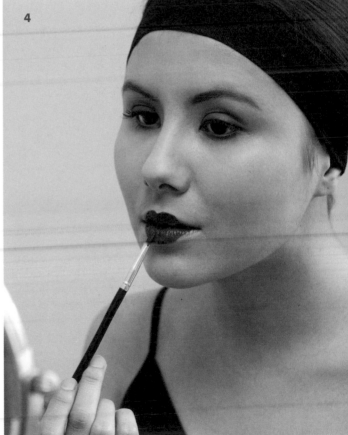

4

*Cupid's-bow lips were a popular look for 'flapper' girls in the 1920s.*

# THE FAUX BOB

*Sleek bobbed haircuts were the height of 1920s fashion. Use the 'faux bob' to sneakily disguise long, flowing locks without having to chop off your tresses.*

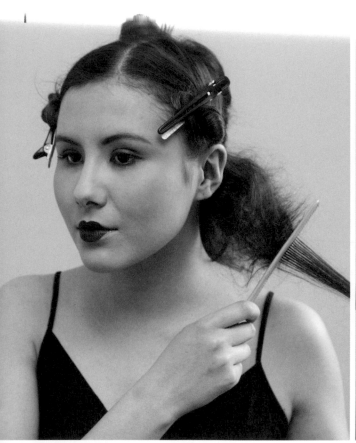

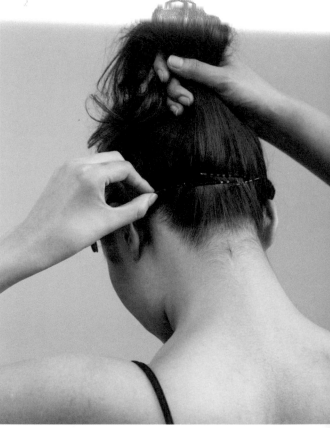

**1** Before styling, set the hair using large heated rollers (see page 14) curling under and taking care to lift the roots. When set, remove the rollers and divide the hair into sections, one on either side of the parting, one at the crown of the head and one at the hairline behind each ear; hold each section in place with section clips. Starting with the sections behind each ear, backcomb the hair very lightly from the roots getting heavier towards the ends of the hair.

**2** Release the section pinned at the crown and gently comb the back section upwards from the roots. Secure the hair with hair grips/bobby pins above nape of the neck, slightly overlapping them in a horizontal line.

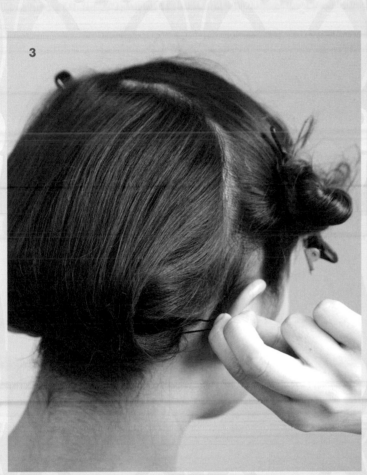

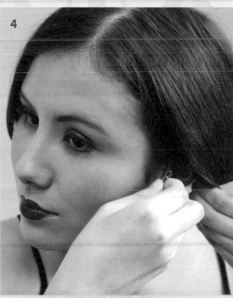

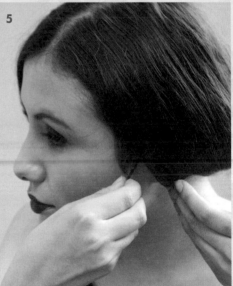

**3** Using your fingers, roll the back section of hair under to create a large roll all across the back of the head. Pin the hair on the inside of the roll to secure it in place.

**4** Take one of the side sections of hair and roll it under across one side of the head. Pin the hair on the inside of the roll under the ear to secure it in place.

**5** Repeat with the other side of the hair, then pin all the way around on the inside of the rolls with hair grips/

bobby pins. Smooth the hair down with a comb so that the bob shape is even all the way around. Finish with a coat of hairspray to achieve a smooth finish.

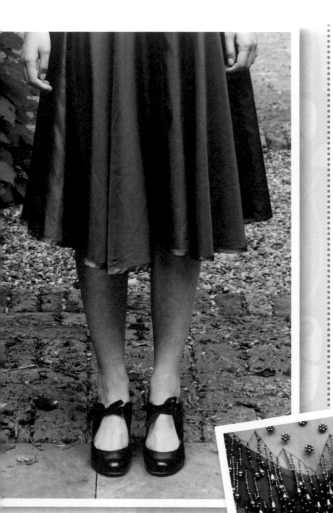

### headbands and hair accessories

The trend for the flat-to-the-head hairstyles that were so on trend at the time can look stunning unadorned and simple; however, they may not be as flattering on round or square face shapes. To complement the hair, try accessorizing with faux tortoiseshell hair combs or slides decorated with pearls or diamantés. 'Flapper'-style headbands with feathers can also give the illusion of slimming the face by adding height.

### capes and boleros

Dresses from the decade were almost always sleeveless, so for ladies who like to cover their arms, try a shoulder cape. Capes and bolero-style jackets were covered with elaborate designs in beads or feathers in the twenties. If purchasing an original falls out of your budget, consider customizing – haberdashery departments/suppliers of notions and specialist bead stores tend to offer a wide range of stock for you to get creative.

### shoes

As the female form began to be exposed by the changes in fashion in the twenties, demand fell on manufacturers to make shoes that revealed the foot and showed off the ankle. The shoe styles synonymous with the twenties are the Mary Jane with its side button fastening and the T-bar – both with a low block heel.

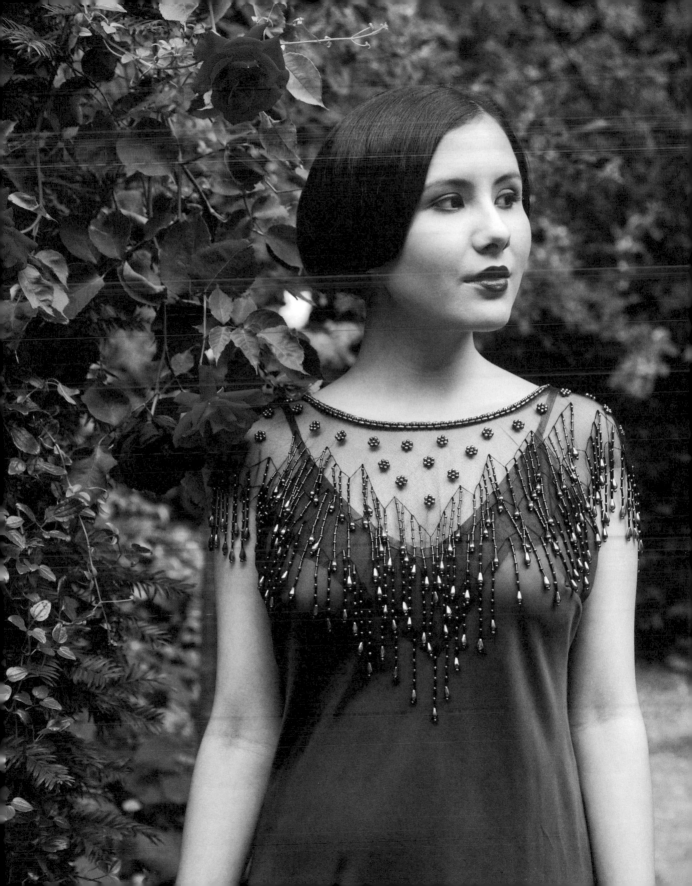

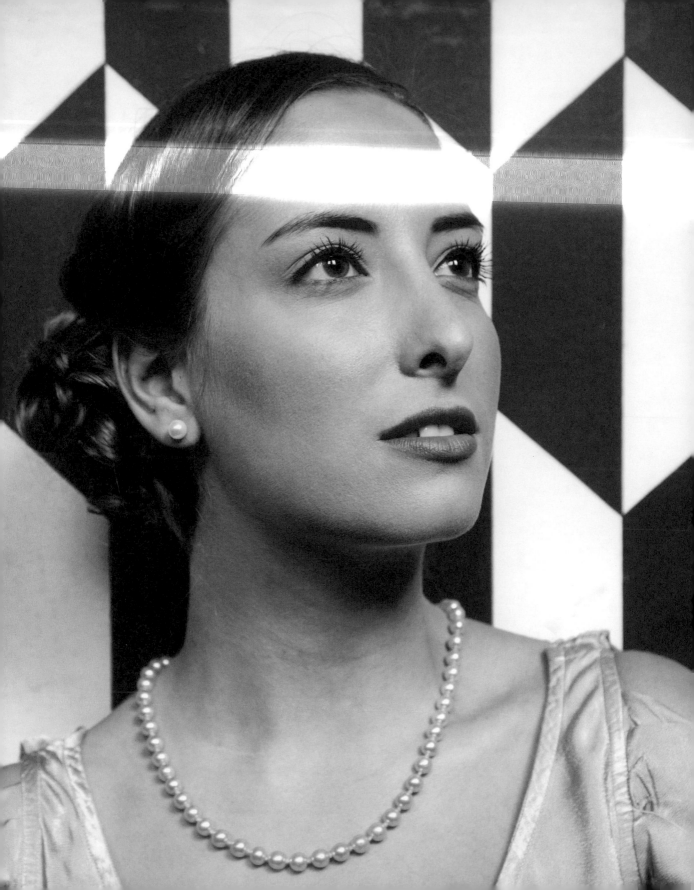

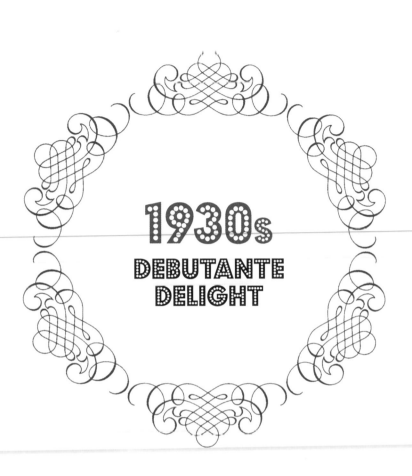

# 1930s
## DEBUTANTE DELIGHT

*The 1930s was the era when women began to look to the glamorous stars of Hollywood for inspiration. With role models such as Jean Harlow and Josephine Baker on the big screen, the period was all about elegance. Great advances were made in the cosmetics industry and lips, eyes, skin and nails were polished to perfection.*

# THE ELEGANT THIRTIES

Having spent the previous few years putting through the Charleston and the Foxtrot, the 'flappers' and 'dandies' of the roaring twenties found themselves in a very different environment when the new decade dawned. Decadence and opulence were a thing of the past as the world fell into economic decline.

In this period of austerity there was no less desire to be beautiful, but times were hard and money was scarce, so women began to think smarter to extend the life of their few luxuries. Vaseline was used to help make eye-shadows and lipsticks go further and shampoo was reserved as a limited necessity.

With stylish actresses such as Joan Blondell, Marlene Dietrich and Olivia De Havilland sporting immaculately coiffured hairs and beautifully made-up faces now seen through advanced Technicolor on the big screen, women sought to re-create the glamour of Hollywood in their own homes with the few products they had access to.

The worlds of beauty and advertising continued their relentless campaign to strive to meet the needs of those women who wanted to emulate the rich and famous, and many new cosmetic products were made available during the decade.

Eye-shadows in a wide range of colours came into use, with shades of blue, green, violet and brown favoured throughout the period. Brows were thin and accentuated with eyebrow pencil.

With advances in film technology, an increased clarity on the big screen meant that actors and actresses demanded better foundation make-up to maintain the appearance of flawless skin – something which remains a concern to this day. As a response to this, Max Factor created the 'Pan-Cake' foundation, which provided a good coverage and soon began being swiped from film sets by stars for use at home. Max Factor seized this opportunity and the product was developed for the retail market in 1937, becoming the fastest and bestselling, single make-up item to date.

For those ladies who were still able to flash a little of their husband's cash, Coco Chanel launched the very first bronzing powder – another product that remains popular to this day. The trendsetting designer had sparked a craze for tanned skin when she had accidently fallen asleep in the sun one afternoon and then attended a society party in the evening. On seeing her tanned complexion and healthy glow, women automatically felt that if Chanel was wearing sun-kissed skin, they all should.

*make-up colour palette:*

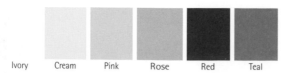

| Ivory | Cream | Pink | Rose | Red | Teal |

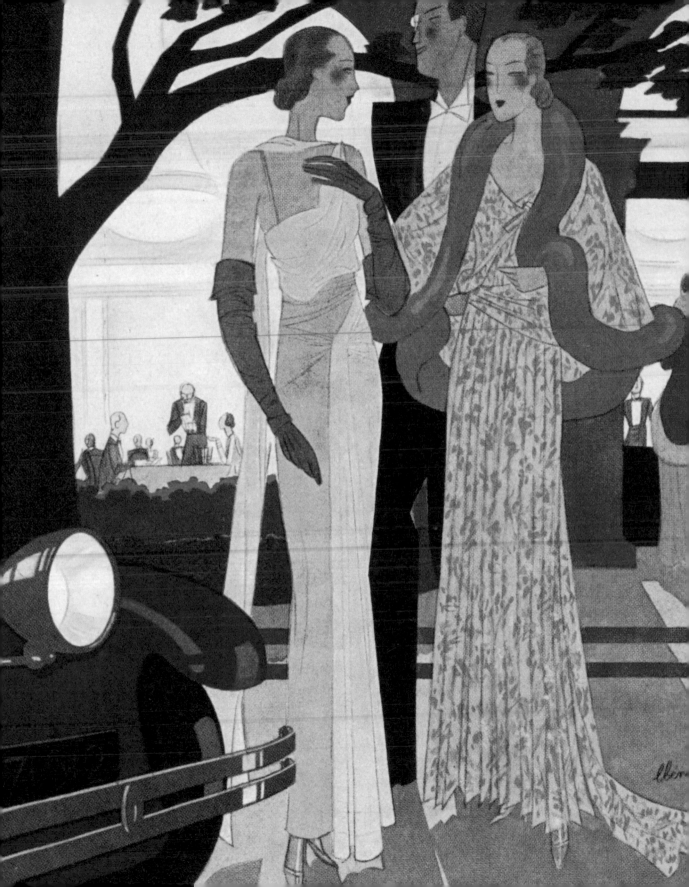

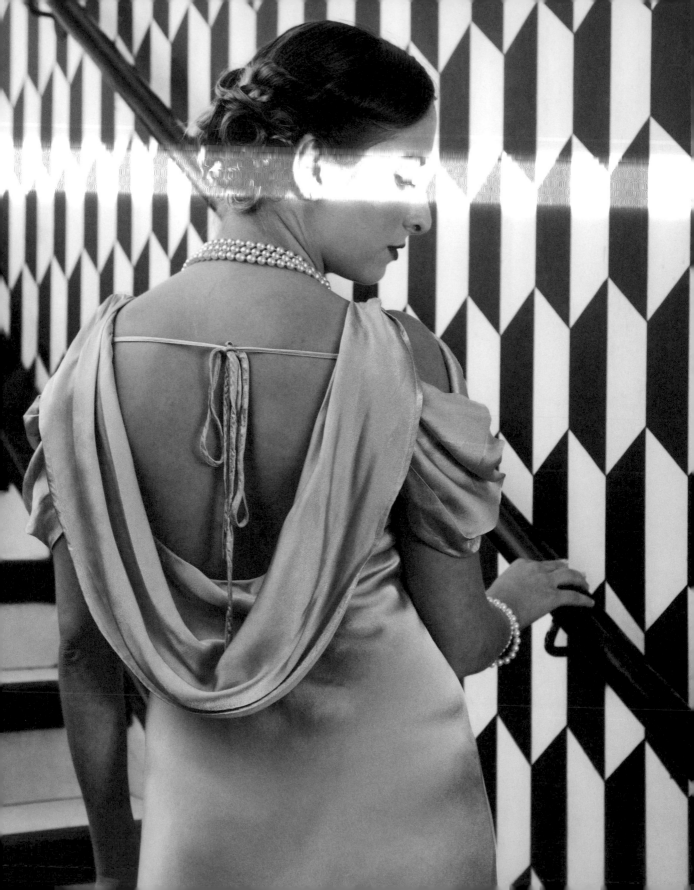

# DEBUTANTE DELIGHT

*In contrast to the frivolity of the 1920s, the following decade favoured simplicity and elegance. Make-up was flawless and used to accentuate the features but remained more natural than in the previous decade.*

Suitable for a formal party or a vintage-style wedding, this typical 1930s accoutrement can be summed up as radiant and timelessly stunning. With advances in the formulation of make-up products such as foundation and blusher during the decade, the focus of this look is on flawless and glowing skin, emulating the looks of the screen sirens of the day.

The cutting edge of occasion fashion in the early part of the decade was incredibly feminine. Shoulders and backs were revealed in floor-skimming evening dresses, which excited designers constructed in ways previously unseen.

In the 1930s, hair was almost always styled off the face in soft waves or in an 'updo' and adorned with clips and combs in marcasite, pearls and other semi-precious jewels. For this look, the hair is swept to one side to frame the face with soft curls pinned up at the nape of the neck to create a chic occasion style that oozes glamour and sophistication. All you need now is an invitation to show off your elegant thirties look.

## TO CREATE THIS LOOK YOU WILL NEED:

### MAKE-UP
Foundation brush ✳ foundation ✳ concealer ✳ translucent powder ✳ round powder brush ✳ round-edged blusher brush ✳ powder blusher in a shade of pink that suits your skin tone

### HAIR
Comb ✳ small heated rollers ✳ clips ✳ hairbrush ✳ hair band ✳ hair grips/bobby pins ✳ hairspray

# GLOWING CHEEKS

*Before applying blusher, prepare your skin with base make-up according to the directions on page 10. Then apply eye make-up according to the directions on page 12, using an eye shadow in a colour of your choice.*

**1** To ensure your blusher has a smooth and even finish, take care to blend in your foundation when applying base make-up, and set with translucent powder. Choose a blusher in a shade of pink appropriate for your skin tone to create a natural, rosy glow.

**2** Sweep a round fluffy brush lightly over and around on your blusher. This will coat the tip of the bristles of the brush and allow for an even distribution of product. Tap excess powder off the brush. This will prevent you applying a heavy and solid block of colour to the cheek area

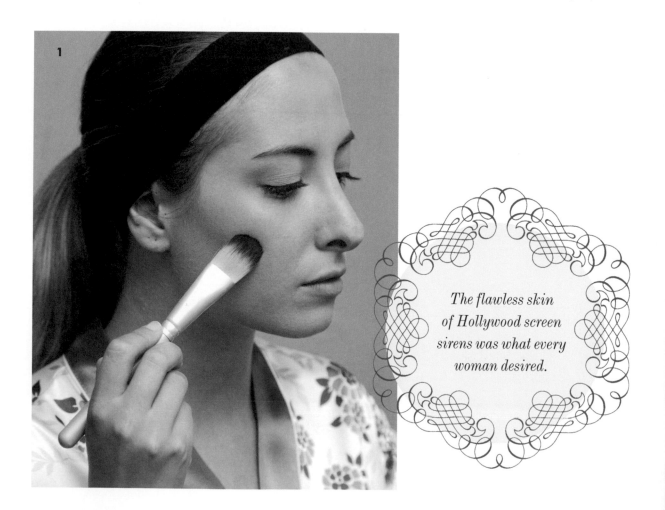

*The flawless skin of Hollywood screen sirens was what every woman desired.*

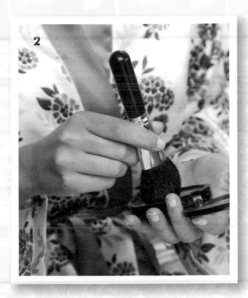

**3** Looking in a mirror, smile until the 'apples' of your cheeks are prominent. This may feel a little strange, but it is important that you study the shape of you face, so that you can use make-up to accentuate your cheekbones and sculpt your face as appropriate.

**4** Apply the blusher in circular motions directly to the apples of your cheeks, gradually moving the blusher brush outwards to blend the edges. Build the intensity of colour as desired by repeating the process

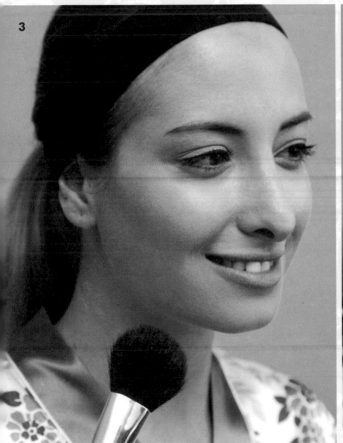

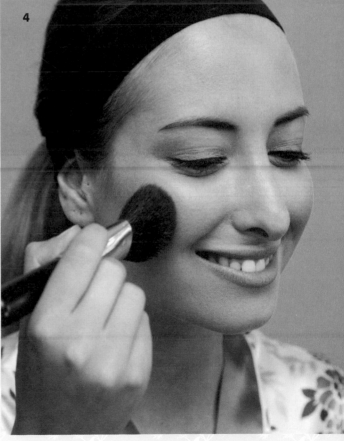

# ELEGANT SIDE BUN

*Setting your hair in heated rollers is the best way to give your hair the shape*
*and movement required for an elegant 'updo' such as this. Heated rollers*

1  Gently comb your hair through and create a side parting. Set your hair using small heated rollers, starting from the side parting and rolling underneath. Secure each roller about 5 cm/2 inches from the root. Leave the hair to set in the rollers, allowing it to cool for at least 10 minutes to ensure that the shape of the curl does not drop.

2  Use a comb to separate off the front section of your hair, maintaining the side parting. Secure the rest of your hair at the back with a clip. Take the heavier side of your side parting, twist it and section it off at the top of your ear and clip it out of the way.

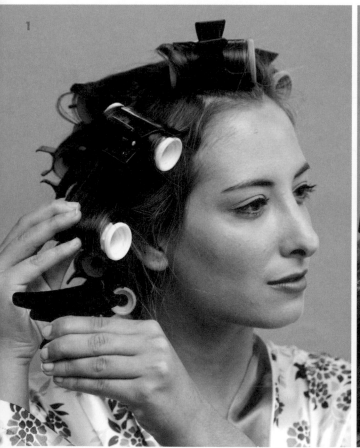

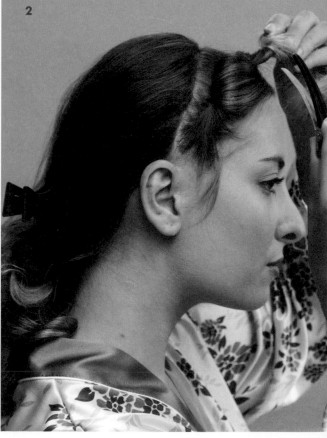

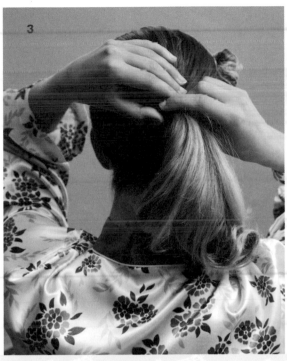

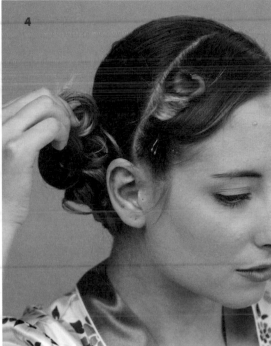

**3** Brush the rest of your hair into a low side ponytail and use a hair band to secure it in place.

**4** Pin the individual curls in your ponytail up to one side at the nape of your neck to create a wavy side bun. Make sure the hair band is not visible and secure the curls with hair grips/bobby pins. You can be as neat or as messy as you choose when pinning your curls, as both options can look very pretty.

**5** Take the sectioned-off front section of your hair and twist it to one side, allowing it to fall softly over your forehead. Pin the end of the section into your bun to complete the look. Add any clips or slides to accessorize your side bun and finish with hairspray.

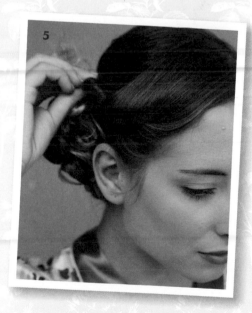

# ACCESSORIZING THIS LOOK
## DEBUTANTE DELIGHT

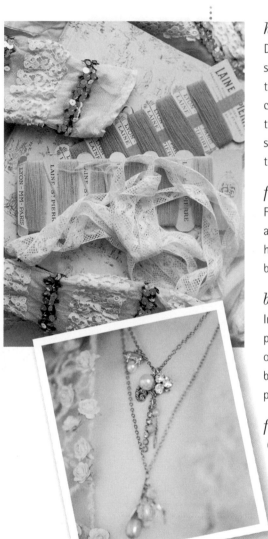

### hats

During the middle of the decade, those wishing to make a statement would elect to wear high-crowned hats, slightly tilted to one side. Individuals with a more modest nature stuck to the cloche hat which is great for oblong or heart-shaped faces, or the trilby, which is better suited to rounder or more square face shapes. These styles are still readily available in mainstream shops today as well as in specialist vintage outlets.

### fur

Fur accessories were immensely popular for those who were still able to afford to own such luxury items. Coats, stoles, wraps and hats, along with fashion trimmings would often be made from beaver, fox, rabbit and mink.

### bags

In general, bags became slightly more utilitarian than in the previous decade. However, it was the 1930s that saw the birth of the much-coveted Hermès saddle bag, later renamed the Kelly bag after the actress Grace Kelly. The accessory is still much prized today.

### fragrance

Complete your look with a spritz of classic thirties fragrance, Elizabeth Arden Blue Grass.

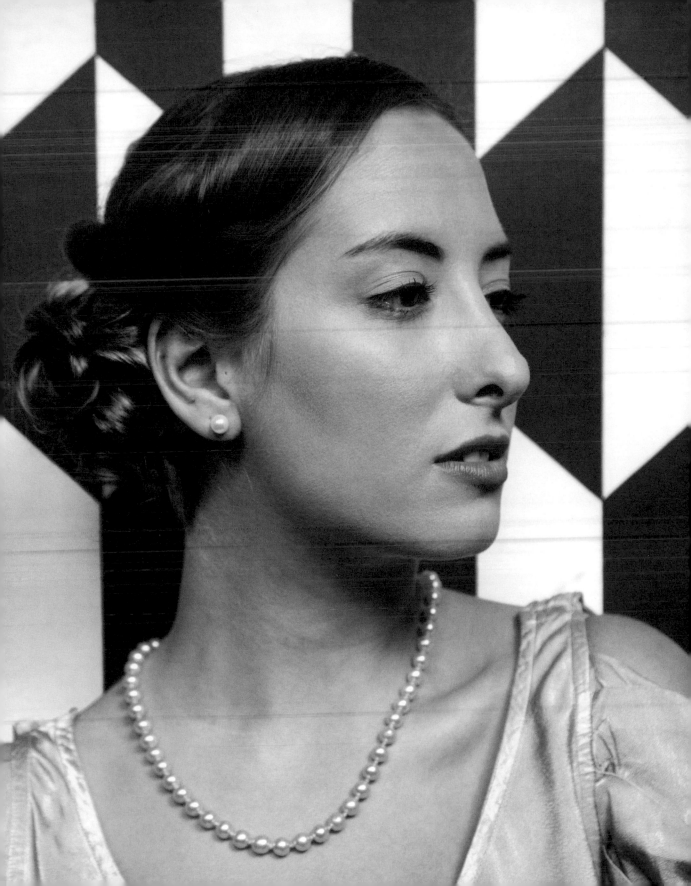

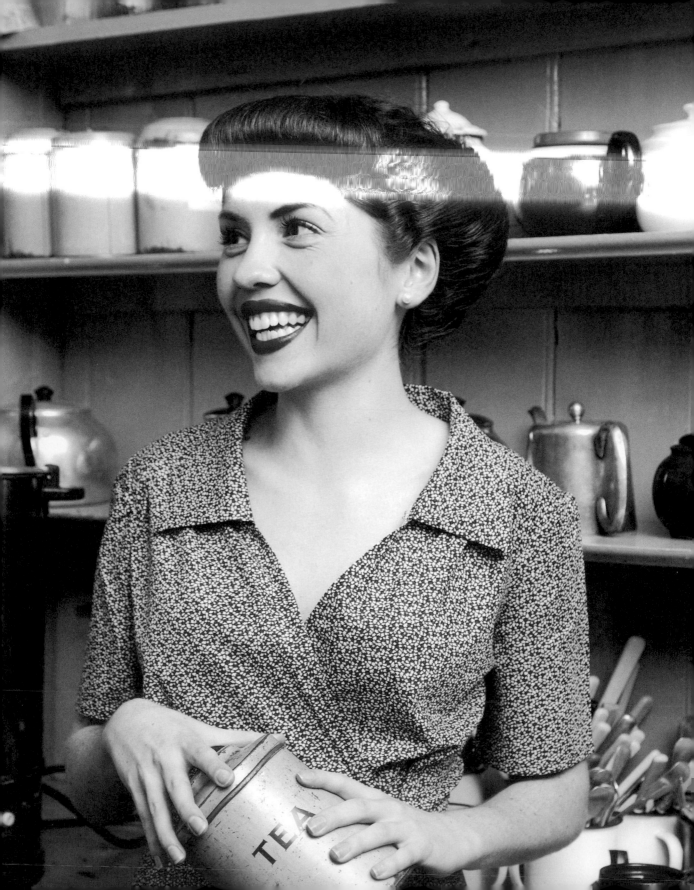

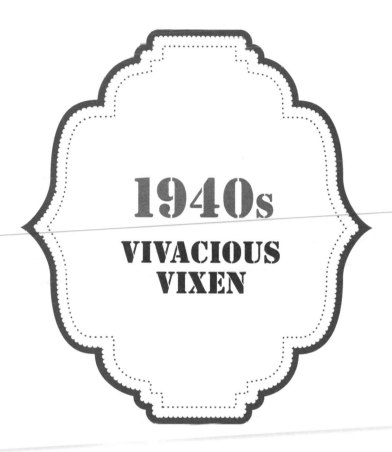

# 1940s

## VIVACIOUS VIXEN

*While there is no denying the hardship that resulted in the wake of World War II, resourcefulness prevailed and many women managed to remain stylish by making do with the few cosmetic products they had. The look was strong and glamorous but not showy, with red lips, bold brows and lashes and a glowing, healthy complexion.*

# THE FRUGAL FORTIES

[...] that most of us take for [...] acceptable for the majority [...] restriction affected all aspects of everyday life. During this period, advertising was awash with ideas, not only for how women should look, but also on how they should conduct themselves to be more attractive. All women's magazines reiterated the mantra that you absolutely had to take pride in your looks and make the most of the few cosmetic products available, because men were in short supply.

As was the case with many other products, lipstick manufacture was hard hit by the war, as key ingredients like castor oil and petroleum were required to be put to a more nationally beneficial use. Elizabeth Arden had created a new magenta shade of lipstick in the early 1940s, but decided that it would be unpatriotic to launch it in the midst of the war and delayed the launch until after the Armistice whistle was blown.

However, red lips in a variety of different shades are essential for an authentic 1940s look, along with glowing skin, achieved by using a slightly darker shade of foundation covered by a lighter powder with a natural, rosy blusher. Eyes were defined with dark brown or black mascara, muted shades of eye-shadow, black eyeliner, and strong, dramatic eyebrows.

To achieve the glowing complexion so highly sought-[...] the [...] your water intake, use [...] liquid or oil-based [...] and avoid any powders containing mica or metallic particles as these were neither available nor fashionable at the time.

The shorter hairstyles made popular in the previous decade were slowly being phased out and replaced by more traditionally 'feminine', flowing styles. Perming solutions were more widely available and hair was often parted to one side and styled in soft curls, victory rolls or in one of several 'updos' that were fashionable at the time.

Women in the services and those who worked in factories considered a perm to be essential as they were required to wear uniforms and so made every effort to express their femininity through their hair and make-up. Straight hair was regarded as most unfashionable and many women chose to have their hair permed or curled their hair with pin curls that they slept in to allow them to set overnight. Another, more economical method of curling hair that was popular during the decade was to rag-roll damp hair and leave it overnight. Hair pomade was used to smooth the hair, create a sleek finish and hold the style in place.

*make-up colour palette:*

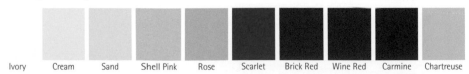

Ivory    Cream    Sand    Shell Pink    Rose    Scarlet    Brick Red    Wine Red    Carmine    Chartreuse

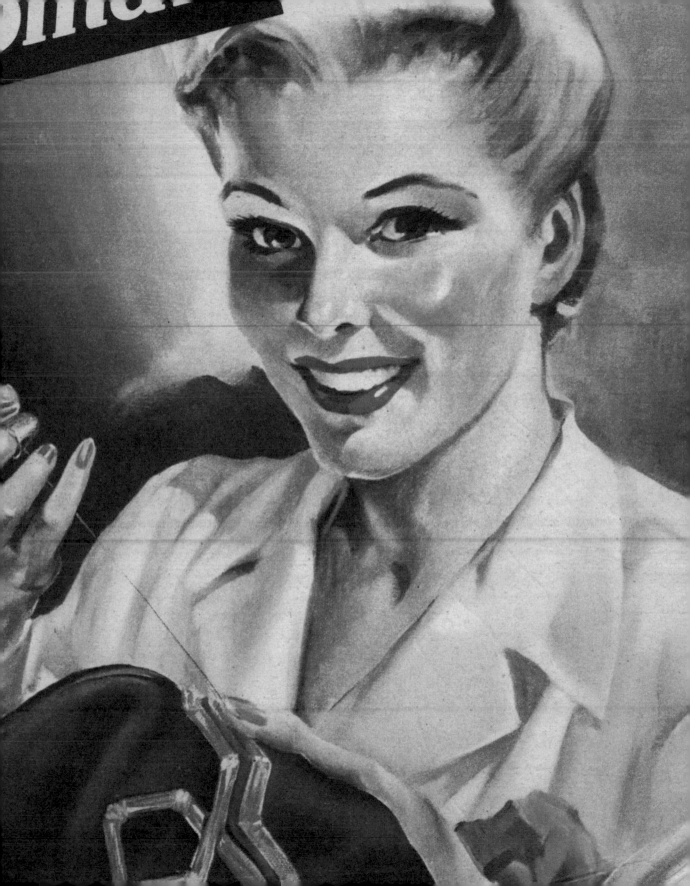

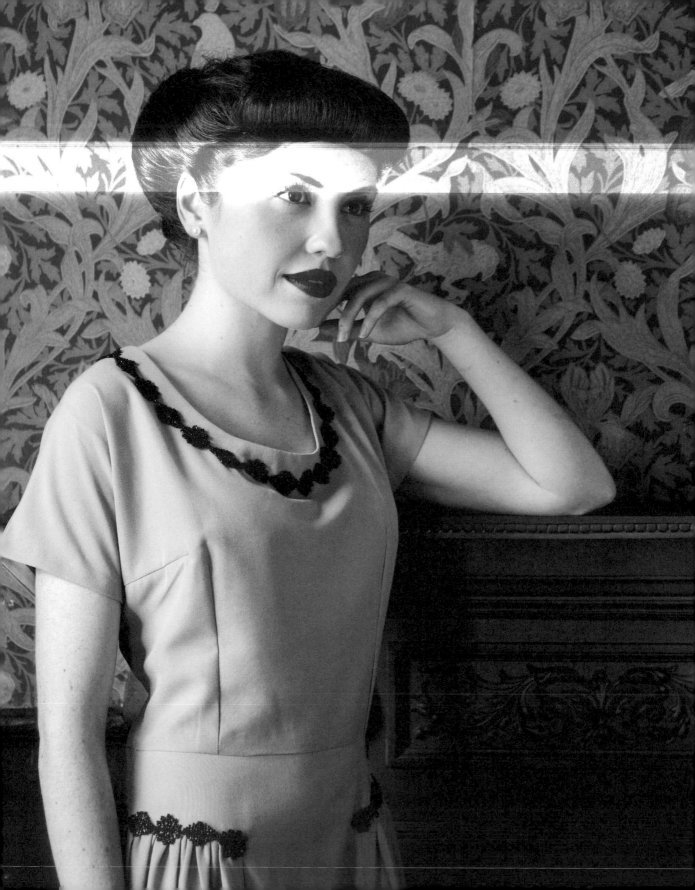

# VIVACIOUS VIXEN

*Austerity just meant the need for a more creative imagination when it came to accentuating your beauty during wartime. This classic 1940s raiment celebrates the understated, feminine style of the period.*

Victory-rolled hair, groomed brows, darkened lashes and kissable full lips are the essential ingredients for this authentic 1940s look, which grew from the desire to appear feminine and attractive using limited resources during wartime. Women used make-up to enhance their natural features, resulting in a timeless, classic beauty.

The impact of World War II meant that there were restrictions on the amount of clothing people could buy and the quantity of fabric manufacturers could use, so fashions were simple and practical. Most women wore knee-length skirts with simply-cut blouses and square-shouldered jackets. Women working for the war effort often wore trousers/pants when the need for efficiency and comfort prevailed.

Elegant but understated, this combination wouldn't look out of place worn for a girls' afternoon lunch, a tea dance or a casual dinner with friends.

## TO CREATE THIS LOOK YOU WILL NEED:

### MAKE-UP
Lip scrub * lip balm * red lip liner * small lip brush * red lipstick * tissue for blotting * clear lip gloss

### HAIR
Fine-tooth comb * sectioning clips * hair grips/bobby pins * hairspray

# LUSCIOUS LIPS

*For an authentic 1940s look, red lips are essential. First, apply a base coat of foundation and blusher acording to the directions on pages 10–11. Choose a red lip shade suited to your skin tone to make the most of this look.*

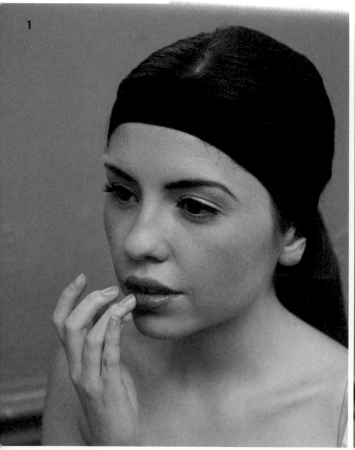

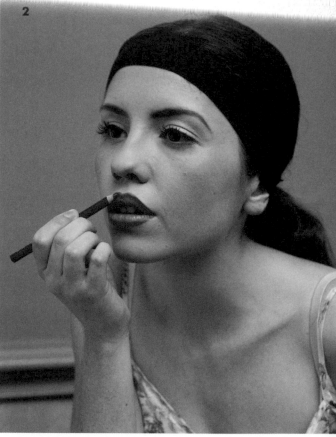

**1** Ensure that your lips are exfoliated and hydrated using a lip scrub and balm. This is especially important around the time that the seasons change, as air conditioning and central heating can leave lips looking and feeling dry. Try and get into a routine of exfoliating your face and lips once or twice a week and moisturizing twice a day
.

**2** Sharpen a red lip liner and slightly blunt the tip on the back of your hand. Wipe the lip liner off your hand with a tissue immediately to avoid any make-up smears on clothes. Line the outer edge of your lips using feathering strokes. This will allow you to correct any imperfections in the natural lip shape and create a symmetrical shape.

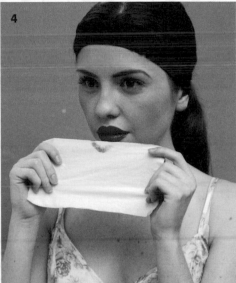

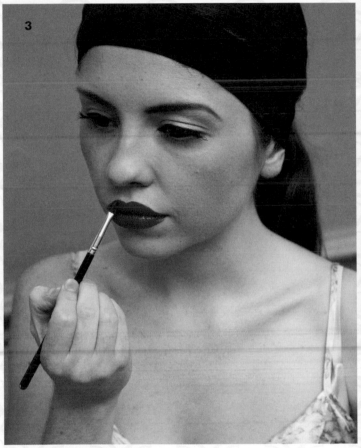

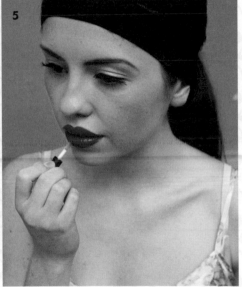

**3** Once you are happy with the symmetry, colour the lip in fully with the liner to act as a base for your lipstick. Apply one coat of lipstick using a small lip brush

**4** Blot your lips with a good quality tissue to avoid fibres sticking to your lips and then apply a second coat of lipstick.

**5** Finish the look by adding a generous coat of clear lip gloss to the centre of the lips to create the illusion of maximum fullness. A good tip is to put a dab of lip gloss on the back of your hand and then apply it to your lips with a lip brush. This avoids the lip colour transferring

# V IS FOR VICTORY ROLLS

*Patriotic victory rolls were at the forefront of 1940s fashion for hair. If you prefer, you can just roll the front section of your hair and leave the rest loose.*

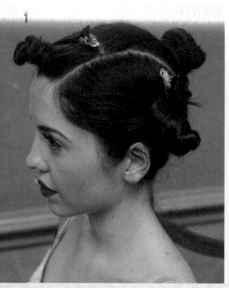
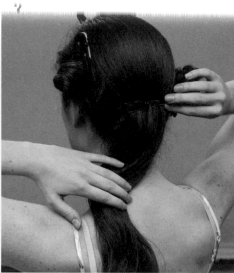
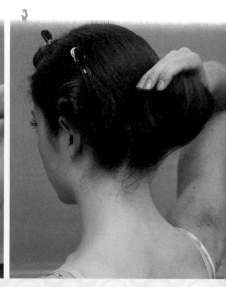

**1** Separate your hair into four sections using the comb. Start by parting your hair on either side about 5 cm/2 inches in from your temples, creating a middle section and two side sections. Twist the two side sections and clip them out of the way on either side of your head. Divide the middle section into two, creating a recangular section from just in front of the crown to your forehead. Twist the front section and clip it out of the way.

**2** Backcomb the back, middle section of your hair gently and place hair grips/bobby pins overlapping horizontally about 2.5–5 cm/1–2 inches above the hairline, depending on how high you want your victory roll to be.

**3** Carefully roll the hair upwards, wrapping it around your fingers to create a roll. Secure the roll with hair grips/bobby pins on the inside of the roll. If you have flyaway hair, spray the section with hairspray before you start rolling it.

**4** Repeat step 2 with both of the two side sections of hair, backcombing each section and inserting hair grips/bobby pins in preparation for rolling.

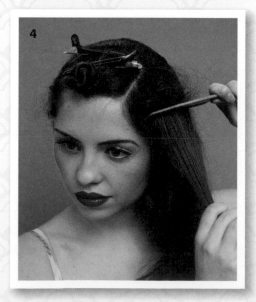

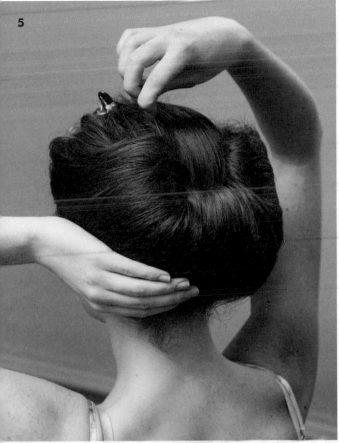
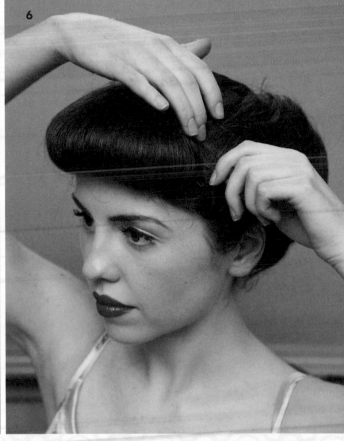

**5** Repeat step 3 with both of the side sections of your hair, rolling the hair inwards and securing the rolls on either side with hair grips inside the roll. Remember to leave space to allow for any hair ornaments or hats that you might consider wearing.

**6** Gently backcomb the front section of your hair. Once again, tame any stray hairs with a light spritz of hairspray and roll the hair under, around your fingers, to create a rolled fringe/bangs effect. Secure the roll with hair grips/bobby pins inside the roll and finish with hairspray.

# ACCESSORIZING THIS LOOK
## VIVACIOUS VIXEN

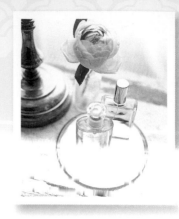

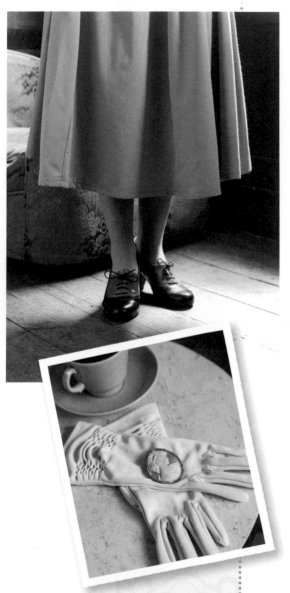

### shoes

Women's shoes underwent a radical change in design at both the beginning and end of the 1940s. Cobblers became inventive when leather was not an option and shoe soles were fashioned from wood and cork. Shoes made from reptile skins were an exotic and highly fashionable statement for any lady, but they were generally only available at high-end retailers with a high-end price tag to match. Block, lavatory and Louis heels were all popular shapes. For authentic forties footwear, look out for original creations from designers of the time, such as Salvatore Ferragamo and Roger Vivier.

### lingerie

It is important to consider what the typical underwear of the time was like when you choose to wear original vintage or contemporary vintage-style clothes, as the undergarments would have shaped the way the clothes hung on the body. Equally, it is important to be aware of your own body shape and to consider what is practical and flattering for your figure.

### fragrance

The longevity of major perfumeries prior to, during and after the war is testament to the importance of scent throughout the twentieth century. The launch of new fragrances during the war years was largely unheard of, but for an authentic wartime aroma, try Muguet des Bois, released by Coty in 1941 or Diorama by Dior from the post-war era – it was launched in 1949.

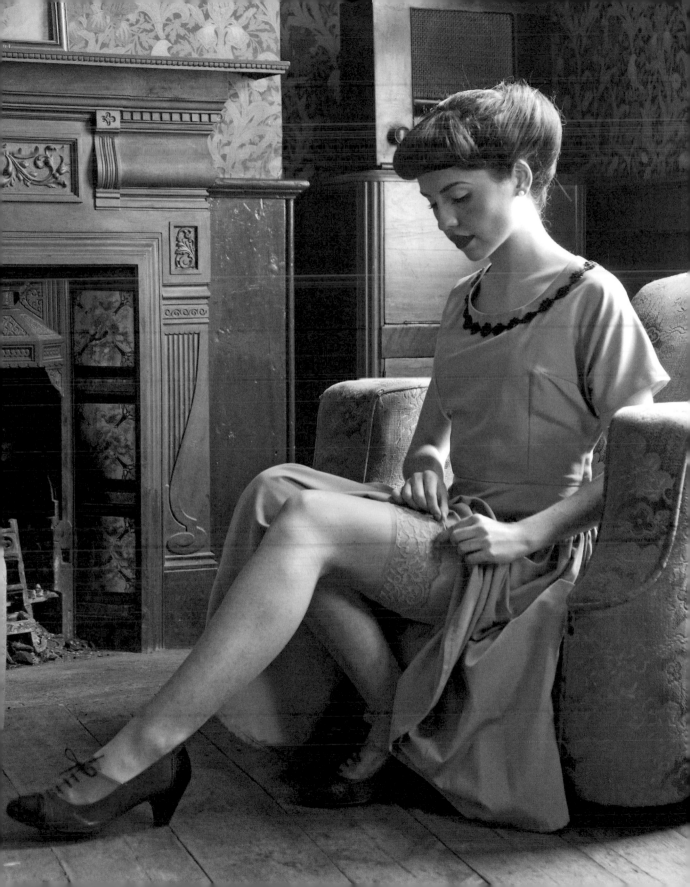

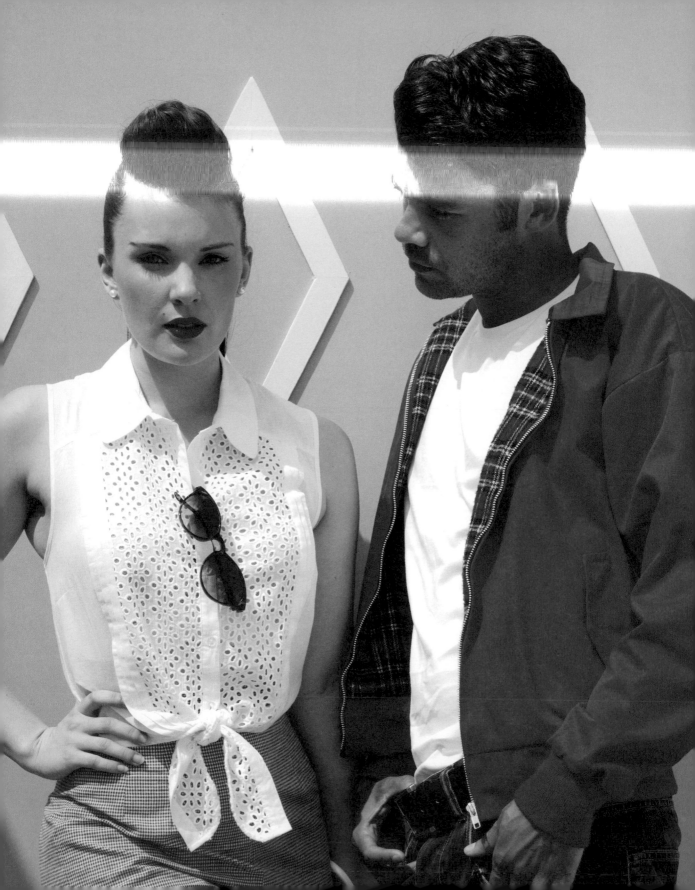

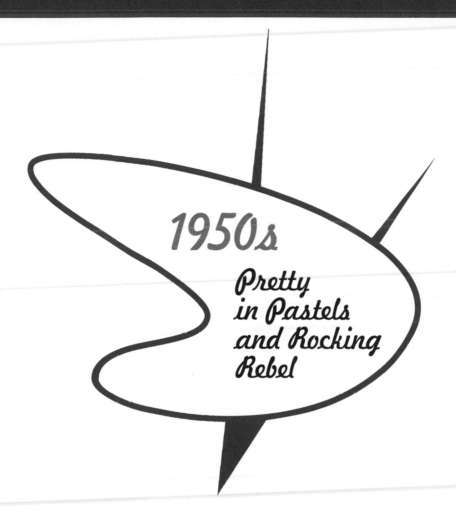

# 1950s

## Pretty in Pastels and Rocking Rebel

*The 1950s was a decade in which style became divided.
Glamorous housewives with perfect pin curls, dressed in
feminine clothes in pretty floral fabrics, are at the heart of
mainstream fifties fashion. In contrast, the rock 'n' roll
youth donned tauntingly tight Capri pants, quiffed their
hair and rocked around the clock to Elvis Presley.*

# The Fabulous Fifties

The shackles of wartime austerity were beginning to loosen in the early years of the 1950s. Peace and prosperity crept over Europe and the utilitarian look of the 1940s was set aside for more glamorous styles, as women were able to embrace the wider range of clothing and cosmetics available.

Fashion in the 1950s was all about celebrating femininity and clothing was designed to enhance a woman's natural curves. Undergarments were sculpted to help create an hourglass figure and bullet bras and high-waisted underwear were worn to create the perfect silhouette. Wiggle dresses and pencil skirts with their nipped-in waists were favoured for their figure-hugging properties. Other popular styles such as jive dresses had full, often pleated skirts, bateau necklines and short sleeves. Wide collars which softened the neckline were also popular. Although dresses and skirts were more common, trousers/pants for women were also becoming popular during this period and fashionable Capri pants were both feminine and practical.

Elvis Presley released 'Heartbreak Hotel' in 1956, giving rise to new hair, make-up and fashion trends among teenagers and young people. A subculture of 'rockers' wore tight sweaters or tie-front blouses with trousers/pants cinched in at the waist and their hair in lofty quiffs and swinging ponytails.

Glamorous celebrities, such as Elizabeth Taylor, Grace Kelly, Bette Davis and Marilyn Monroe, were extremely influential on style trends. Neatly-tinted eye-shadow, lashings of mascara and strong, flicked eyeliner framed by perfectly-groomed brows remained the look preferred by many. Blusher in varying hues of magenta and pink, was typically positioned high on the face to lift the cheekbones, whilst lips were perfectly lined and finished in a sultry shade of red. The range of lipsticks in pastel colours started to increase around 1956. These colours became especially popular among young women as they were perceived as being less sexually evocative. By the end of the decade, developments in the cosmetics industry gave rise to the addition of titanium to lipstick formulations, creating new frosted shades that remained highly fashionable well into the 1960s.

Hair trends dictated soft feminine curls throughout the decade – though variations of length were acceptable. Short hair was often permed or fashioned into a poodle cut. Mid-length or long hair was sometimes accessorized with a headscarf. If you couldn't afford a visit to the salon, there was an abundance of instructions for home hairstyling in every woman's weekly magazine, and pins and rollers were standard equipment for every self-respecting woman's hairstyling regime.

*make-up colour palette:*

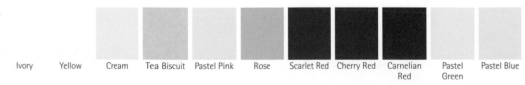

| Ivory | Yellow | Cream | Tea Biscuit | Pastel Pink | Rose | Scarlet Red | Cherry Red | Carnelian Red | Pastel Green | Pastel Blue |

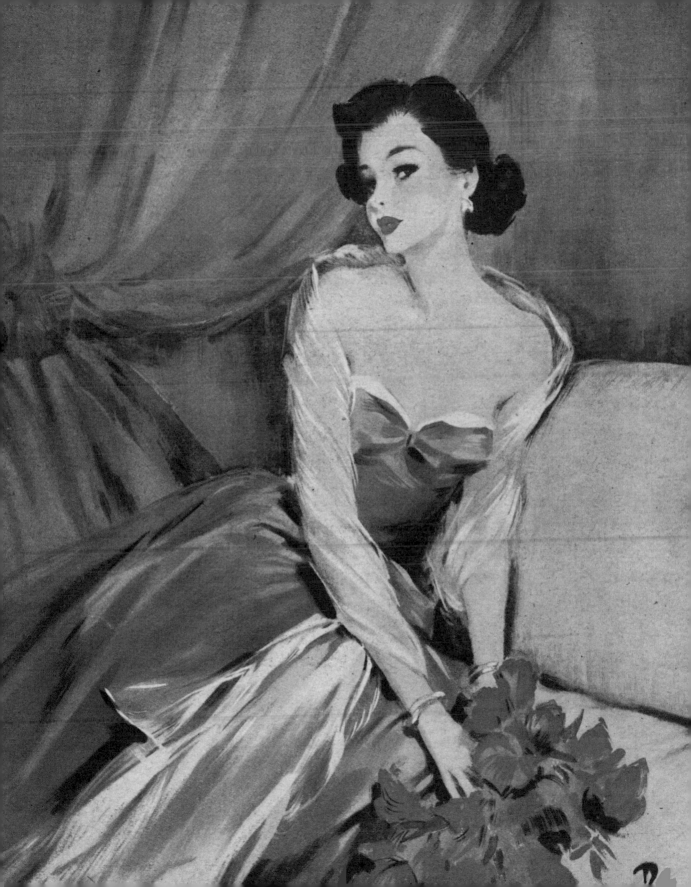

# Pretty in Pastels

*The archetypal 1950s housewife cut a glamorous figure with her immaculate hair and fresh-faced radiance. This look is influenced by the American fashion seen predominantly in the early years of the decade.*

This pretty-as-a picture ensemble is perfect for a family lunch or an afternoon tea party. Get out your best tea dress in a feminine floral print or pastel colour and accessorize with a simple and elegant string of pearls.

The emphasis of fashion in the 1950s was feminity, so wear a pale shade of eye-shadow, barely there eyeliner and a defining mascara to fan out your lashes. Make sure eyebrows are groomed and filled in for definition. Choose a pastel colour lipstick and a blusher in a rose-tinted hue to give your cheeks a pretty flush.

Hairstyles throughout the 1950s were well-groomed and stylish, so finish the look by dressing your hair in soft curls with additional rolls pinned around your face.

## To create this look you will need:

### Make-up
Small, angled brush ✳ matte brown or black brow powder or eye-shadow ✳ brow comb ✳ brown or black eyebrow pencil ✳ cotton bud/Q-tip ✳ eye make-up remover

### Hair
Heated rollers ✳ hairbrush ✳ fine-tooth comb ✳ hair grips/bobby pins ✳ hairspray

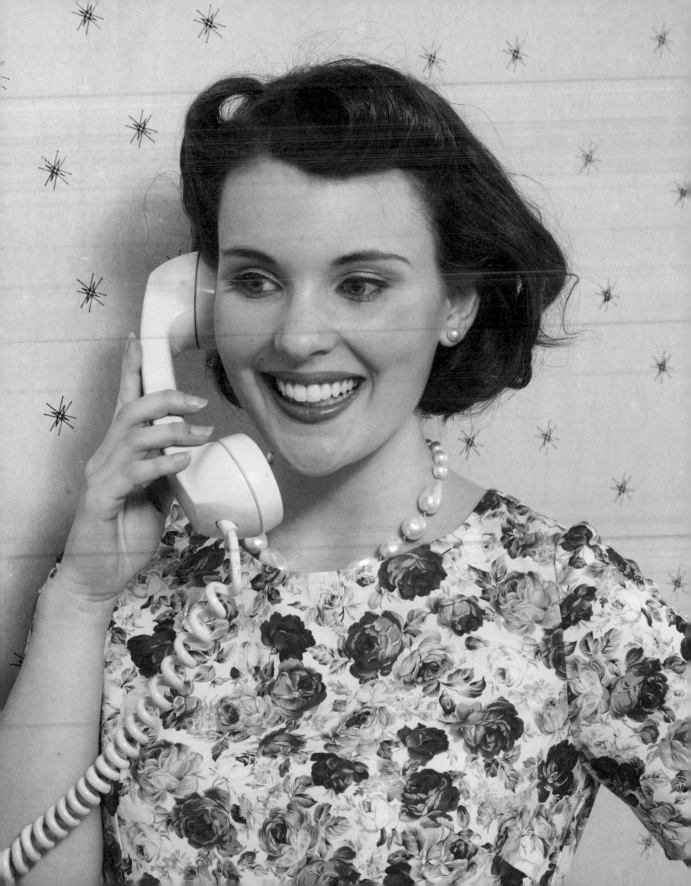

# Beautiful Brows

*For an authentic 1950s look, well-groomed eyebrows are essential. Try to match the colour of your brow powder to the natural colour of your eyebrows.*

1 Using a brow brush or a fine-tipped brush loaded with a brow powder, apply the colour to match the natural colour of your eyebrows starting from the inner part of your brow. Build the colour gradually, running the colour all the way through the length of your natural brow.

2 After applying colour to both eyebrows, brush through with an eyebrow comb. Use the eyebrow comb to shape the brow in an upward direction, making sure it is evenly distributed all the way through the natural length of your eyebrows.

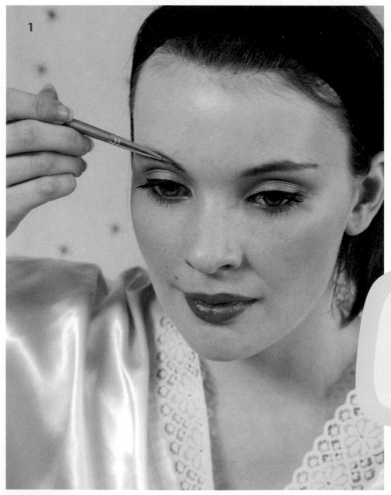

*Neatly shaped and well-groomed eyebrows act as a frame for your features.*

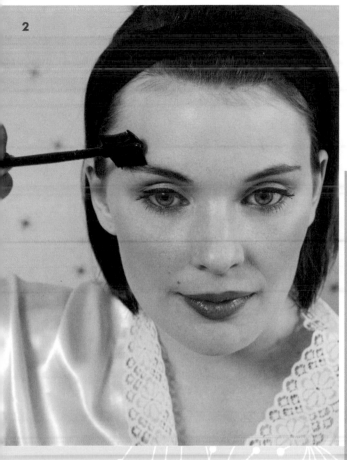

2

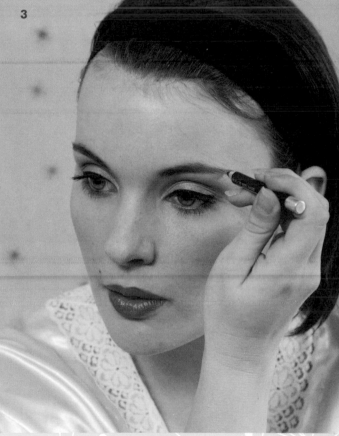

3

**3** Using a sharpened eyebrow pencil, extend the length of the outer section of each of your eyebrows in a downwards movement. Use short, feathery strokes for the most natural effect and layer the brows to a soft point. Don't extend the brows too far, or it will look unnatural

**4** Dip a cotton bud/Q-tip in a small amount of eye make-up remover and gently clean around the edges of your eyebrows to ensure they are neat.

# Delicate Curls

*This versatile fifties hairstyle looks great on mid-length or long hair. If your hair is freshly-washed, apply a generous amount of volumizing mousse to the medium-sized hair in rollers. This will enhance the life of your curls.*

1 Brush the hair, then use a comb to create a side parting. Set the hair using heated rollers, starting from the parting and moving down towards the hairline. Scale down the size of the rollers from large to small as you work towards the base of the neck.

2 After leaving the rollers to set for about 10 minutes, remove all the rollers and re-create the original side parting.

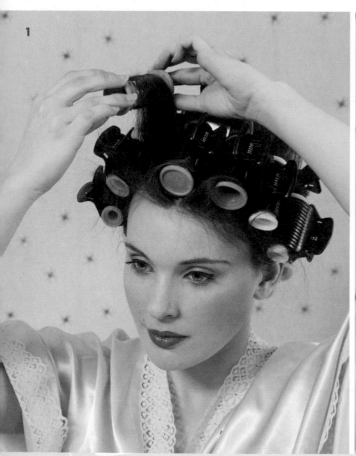

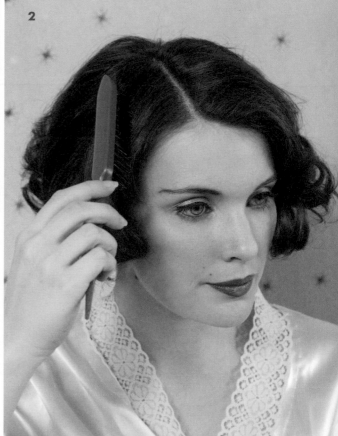

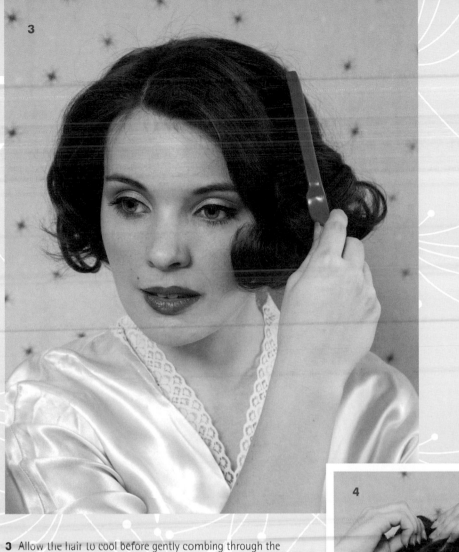

3

**3** Allow the hair to cool before gently combing through the curls to create a soft wave effect.

**4** To create rolls at the front of your hair, backcomb the sections on either side of your parting. Placing your fingers on your scalp where you want the first roll to be positioned, roll the hair over your fingers and pin the hair in place with hair grips/bobby pins on the inside of the roll. Repeat on the other side and finish with hairspray.

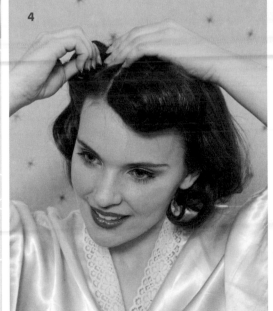

4

# Accessorizing This Look
## Pretty in Pastels

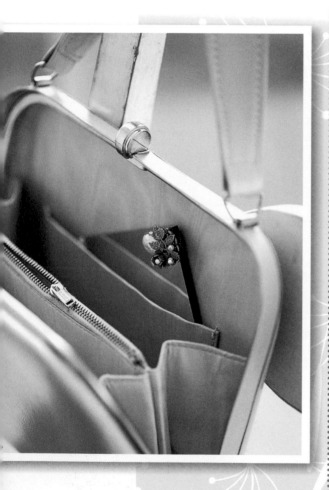

### hats

If you want to complete an authentic 1950s outfit, don't forget your hat. Look out for tri-corner ensembles with pretty embellishments, Juliet caps and berets. Famous milliners of the time include John P. John, Paulette, Gilbert Orcel and Lilly Daché.

### bags

The development of thermoplastics during the postwar years led to the creation of Lucite and the birth of the Lucite bag. These bags were mass produced in a variety of colours and designs. They were carried by girls and ladies of all ages and are much coveted today as works of art.

### lingerie

The hourglass figure of the 1950s owes everything to underwear. High-waisted knickers/panties will nip and tuck your stomach perfectly. Bras were ultra-supportive in the1950s and the famous bullet bra was designed in a conical shape without wires to lift and enhance the bust, creating that iconic 'pointy' shape.

### fragrance

Dior manufactures Diorissimo (1956), a great day perfume with floral notes, as well as the zesty, citrus Eau Fraîche (1953), which works well as a summer scent. The signature scent of the decade has to be Estée Lauder's Youth-Dew (1954) – a sumptuously rich, earthy, almost powdery evening scent best suited to autumn or winter.

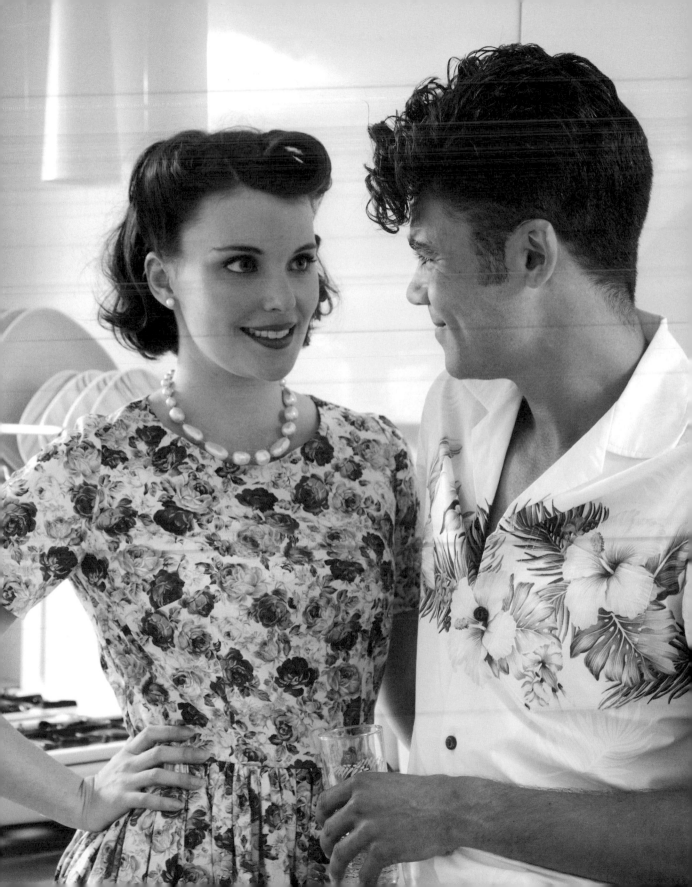

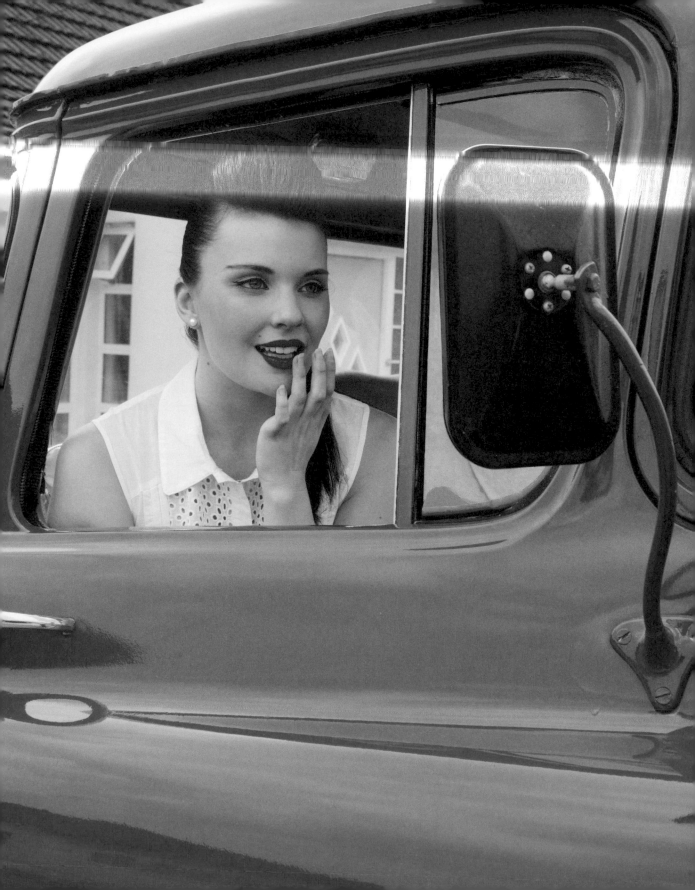

# Rocking Rebel

*The youth of the 1950s cried out for change within the beauty and fashion markets. With subcultures such as 'rockers' and 'teddy boys' emerging, trends became edgier and more alternative than ever before.*

Best suited to a casual occasion such as a trip to the bowling alley with friends, or an evening watching your favourite band, this 1950s 'rocker' look is fun and feisty. Don your tightest pair of Capri pants, tease your quiff to the highest proportions and prepare to crank up the sounds of Elvis while you rock 'n' roll the night away.

Eye-shadow colour preference varied, but the new, sexy 'rocker' look involved accentuating the size and shape of the eye with liquid liner dramatically flicked out to the sides. Worn with a neutral or light shade of eye-shadow and volumising mascara, this bold eye make-up style is guaranteed to make a statement.

To re-create this classic look, lipstick must be red but take your time finding the shade that is most flattering for your complexion. Generally, reds with blue undertones suit skin tones that have a pink hue, and orange tones suit warmer, more yellow and olive skin tones. For the ultimate fifties finishing touch, use a kohl eyeliner pencil to add a 'beauty spot'.

## To create this look you will need:

### Make-up
Neutral eye-shadow ✳ eye-shadow brush ✳ Thin eyeliner brush ✳ black liquid eyeliner ✳ cotton bud/Q-tip ✳ eye make-up remover

### Hair
Section clips ✳ fine-tooth comb ✳ hair brush ✳ hair band ✳ hair extension (optional) ✳ hair grips/bobby pins ✳ hairspray

# Bold Eyeliner

*To create the bold, sexy eye make-up style of the 'rockers', apply eye-shadow in a neutral colour all over your eye sockets before applying your eyeliner.*

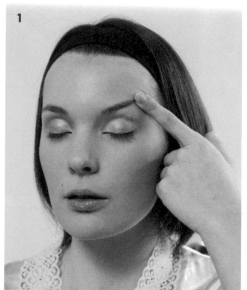

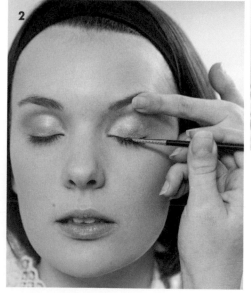

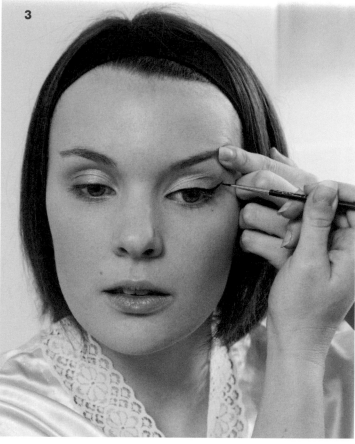

**1** Study the shape of your eyes and your brows. This will help you determine where you should position your eyeliner flick. Gently lift the outer end of your eyebrow to flatten and stretch the skin of the eye socket. This will help you to draw an even line.

**2** Line your eyelids with liquid eyeliner, positioning the eyeliner brush flat against your lash line ¾ of the way in from the outer edge. Stay as close to your natural lash line as possible for the best density of colour.

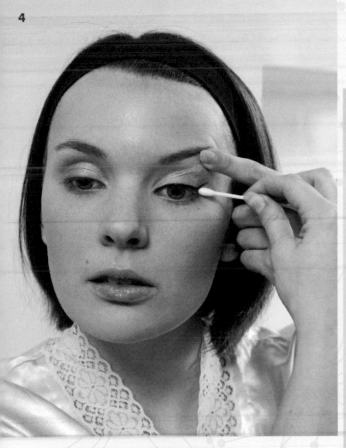

**4**

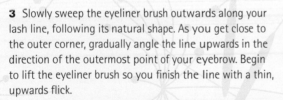

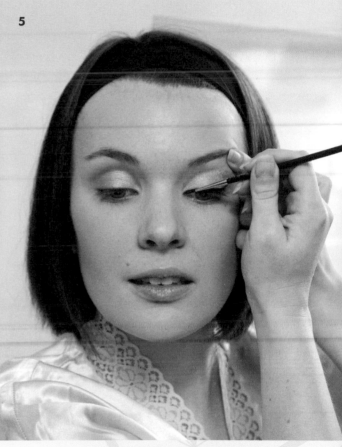

**5**

**3** Slowly sweep the eyeliner brush outwards along your lash line, following its natural shape. As you get close to the outer corner, gradually angle the line upwards in the direction of the outermost point of your eyebrow. Begin to lift the eyeliner brush so you finish the line with a thin, upwards flick.

**4** If you wish to correct the angle of the flick, dip a cotton bud/Q-tip in a small amount of eye make-up remover and sweep it upwards, starting at the base of the outer corner of your eye, to remove any imperfections.

**5** Finish your eyeliner by lining the inner corners of your eyes using the very tip of your eyeliner brush. Starting at the innermost corner of your eyes, with your brush positioned as close to your lash line as you can and sweep your eyeliner brush outwards to create a full and solid line.

# Ponytail with Quiff

*You don't have to have long hair to have a swinging 1950s-style ponytail. Use a hair extension in the same colour as your hair to create the illusion of length.*

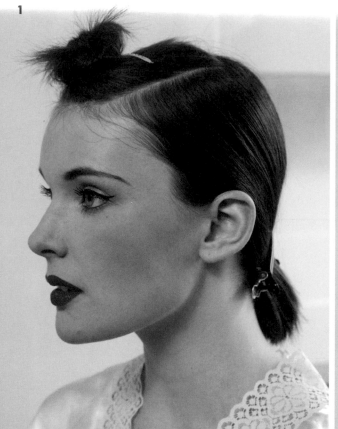

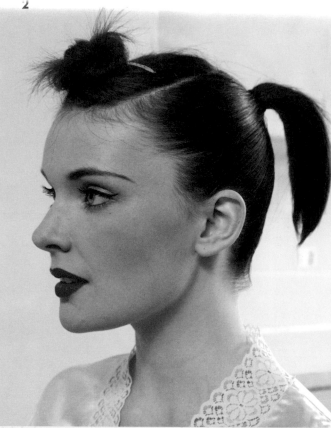

**1** Take a rectangular section of your hair from your temples to your crown and clip it out of the way with a section clip. This section of hair will be used to create your quiff.

**2** Brush the rest of your hair upwards into a ponytail and secure with a hair band. Make sure the ponytail is sitting near the crown of your head to create height.

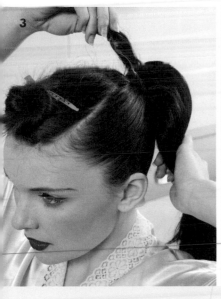

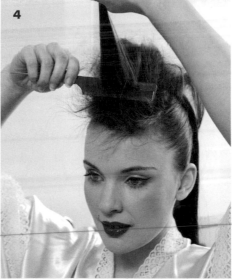

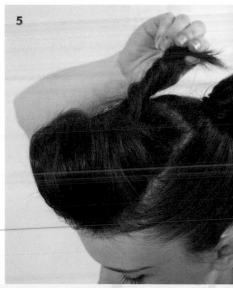

**3** If you have short hair and are using a hair extension, clip in the hair extension and wrap it around the ponytail. Arrange the extension so that it blends in with your natural hair and sits appropriately in your ponytail.

**4** Gently backcomb the front rectangular section of your hair with a fine-tooth comb.

**5** Once you have backcombed the front section, gently smooth the backcombed hair into a mini ponytail. Twist the bottom of the mini ponytail and push it forward to create height. How far you push it forward will determine how high your quiff will be. Once you are happy with the height, secure the twisted section with hair grips/bobby pins to hold your quiff in place.

**6** Tuck any stray hair from your quiff into your ponytail, then pin any stray ends out of the way and smooth with a comb. And, as an additional finishing touch, wrap a small

section of hair around the hair band to conceal it and secure with a single hair grip/bobby pin. Spritz with hairspray for long-lasting hold.

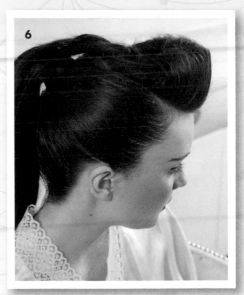

# Accessorizing This Look
## Rocking Rebel

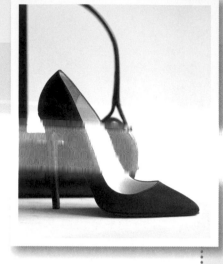

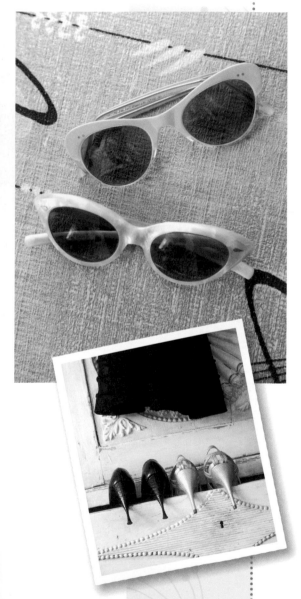

### shoes

After the wide success of Christian Dior's New Look in the late 1940s, Roger Vivier began working closely with Dior in 1953 and gave new life to a design that was first introduced in the previous century – the stiletto. Although women had been known to wear a version of what we refer to as a stiletto as far back as Victorian times, the required technology to produce a stable, thin, high heel had not been mastered until midway through the decade. Mehmet Kurdash launched a range of designs under the brand name Gina in 1954, naming the company as a tribute to his favourite actress, Gina Lollobrigida. Gina shoes have continued to be worn by celebrities and royalty to this day. Girlie girls should consider peep toes, kitten heels, winklepickers and slingbacks, whilst those seeking more practical footwear can opt for creepers, saddle shoes and rock 'n' roll favourites: Converse trainers/sneakers.

### spectacles

The favoured shape for spectacles in the 1950s favoured the 'cats eye', which is very distinct. Original retro frames were often glittery or adorned with diamantés and made quite a statement. Many modern stockists offer both plain lense frames and sunglasses as an alternative.

### scarves

Worn around the head, scarves would be tied to form a small bow on top, often positioned just behind the quiff. They were also worn around the neck. Patterns on scarves would vary but traditional paisley bandanas were often worn by 'rockers' or 'teddy girls'.

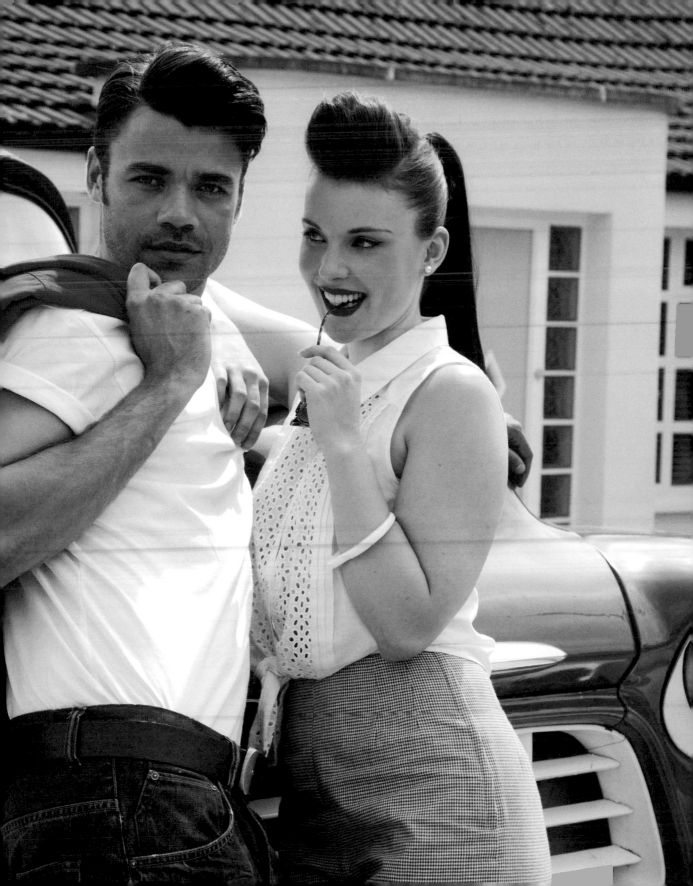

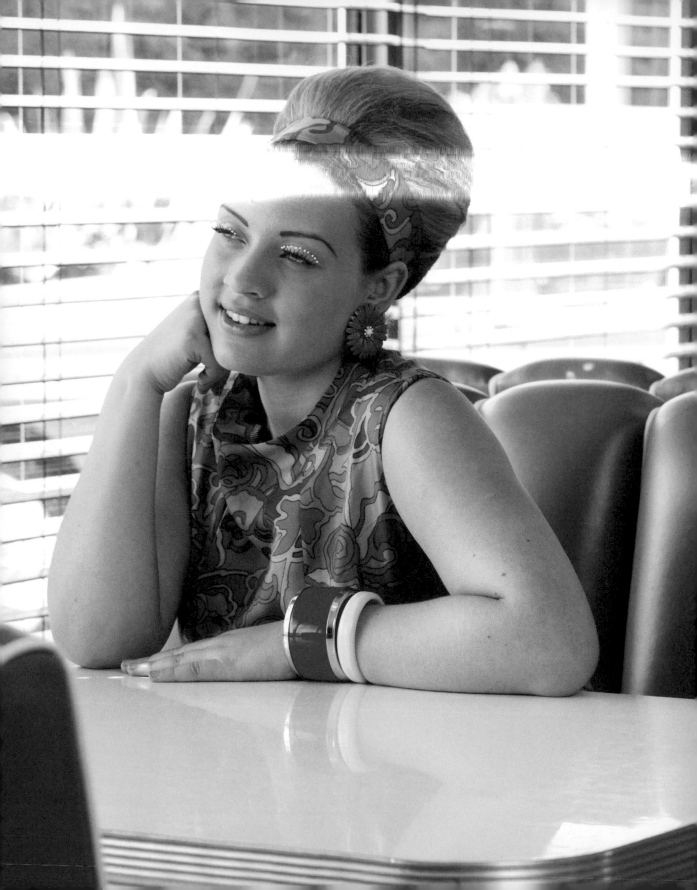

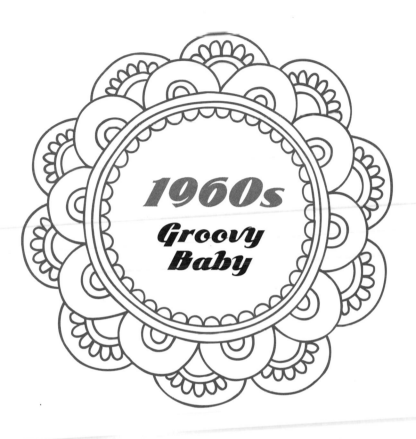

# 1960s

## Groovy Baby

A colourful era unfolded during the 1960s, as women began
to embrace new-found freedom and reject the demure
styles of the 1950s in favour of a more playful approach
to fashion and beauty. Make-up was all about the eyes,
which were emphasized with dramatic colours and false
lashes, while lips were played down with soft nudes.

# The Swinging Sixties

The halcyon postwar experience drew to an abrupt end as the clock ticked into the 1960s. It was a decade that was to see the assassinations of JFK and Martin Luther King, in 1963 and 1968 respectively, and the death, in 1962, of Hollywood bombshell Marilyn Monroe, who was laid to rest in a dress by her favourite designer, Emilio Pucci.

Women had long been fighting an arduous battle for equality in the workplace and the modern feminist movement was building strength to change how women were perceived in every aspect of society. Demand to not be objectified and liberation from the kitchen sink was what many strived to achieve with a new wave of contemporary thinking.

Licensed birth control facilitated previously unprecedented sexual freedom, which served to dictate a groundbreaking change in fashion. Women no longer conformed to the delicate, subservient label that was previously bestowed upon them; now they were burning their bras and demanding change.

It is probably fair to say that chemical consumption played a huge part in the evolution of fashion throughout the decade, resulting in radical alterations to make-up and hair trends that became synonymous with the swinging sixties. The new beauty aesthetic was in stark contrast to the chic elegance that had preceded it. Faking it also became fashionable, with peroxide, false lashes, and cosmetic enhancement becoming a consideration even for the girl next door.

Hairstyles and colour trends altered at a fast pace. Dye from Miss Clairol had hit the shelves in 1956 and rapidly grew in popularity, giving women the flexibility not only to cover emerging grey, but also to adopt an entirely new look whenever the mood took them – all this AND from home. Curls fell from favour around 1963 and were replaced by straight, centre-parted locks, which became a defining style of the 'hippies' towards the end of the decade. Backcombing and flicked ends were the staple style for many, until the ultra-slim model, Twiggy, burst onto the fashion stage with a platinum-blonde pixie cut, Bambi-esque monochrome eyes and nude lips.

Youth subculture, the modernists or 'mods', as they became commonly known, embraced the elfin teenager as a female fashion icon and adopted London's Carnaby Street as their 'office'. Mods were forward-thinking fashionistas, heavily influenced by the Continent – Italy, in particular. The 'Mod Princess' and hairdresser Vidal Sassoon can both be thanked for the popularity of short, sculpted hairstyles and held partly responsible for making hats a casualty of the decade; they were, in any case, becoming disregarded as everyday wear due to the increasing trend for casual dress.

*make-up colour palette:*

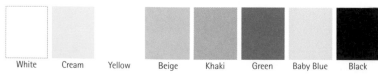

White    Cream    Yellow    Beige    Khaki    Green    Baby Blue    Black

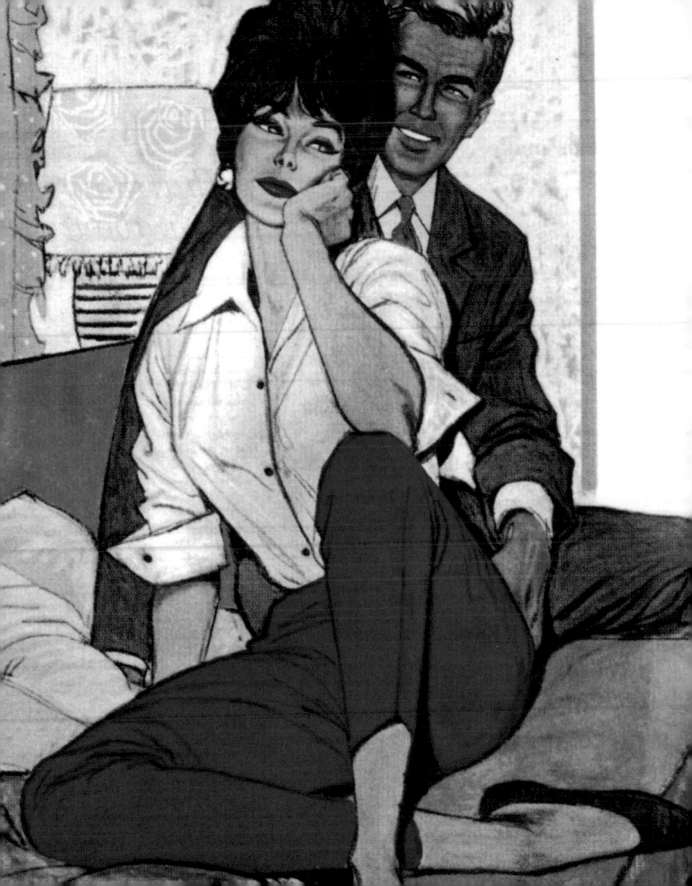

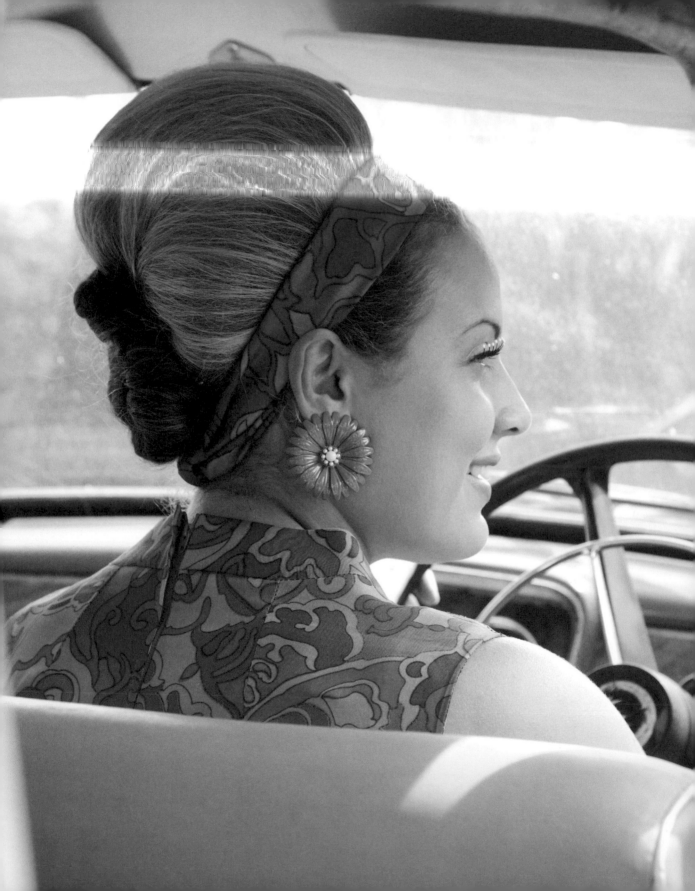

# Groovy Baby

*This iconic 1960s look goes hand in hand with the vibrancy of psychedelic fashion and is a classic example of the creative and artistic hair and make-up designs seen throughout the decade.*

For ladies unwilling to part with their long locks, there was the 'beehive', also known as the 'B-52' due to its resemblance to the nose of the B-52 Bomber. Created by hairstylist Margaret Vinci Heldt, the beehive was designed to hold its shape and was modelled on a fez-like hat that she owned. Elegant and sophisticated, it was an ideal hairstyle for both work and play. Big hairstyles were a popular choice in general and required quantities of industrial-strength lacquer to tame them, so it is no surprise that by 1964 hairspray had become the biggest-selling beauty product in the marketplace.

White eye-shadow was a popular choice. Worn with a contrasting colour in the socket line to add depth and definition, and exuberant false lashes to add drama, it really works to brighten and show off the eyes. For an authentic 1960s look that is guaranteed to turn heads, complement the bold eyes with a flawless matte base with a very gentle hue of colour on the cheeks to contour the face and a nude shade on the lips, which won't steal any of the limelight from the eyes.

## To create this look you will need:

### Make-up
Brow and lash comb ✳ brow pencil or powder ✳ medium and small eye-shadow brushes ✳ white eye-shadow ✳ blue eye-shadow ✳ false lashes and lash glue ✳ tweezers ✳ black mascara

### Hair
Hairbrush (a Tangle Teezer is ideal) ✳ pin-tail comb ✳ sectioning clip ✳ hair donut ✳ hair pins or hair grips/bobby pins ✳ hairspray

# Spectacular Lashes

*False lashes will transform your look in a blink and come in many different styles, from subtle individual or corner lashes that give a natural effect to dramatic looks embellished with crystals and feathers for a playful vibe.*

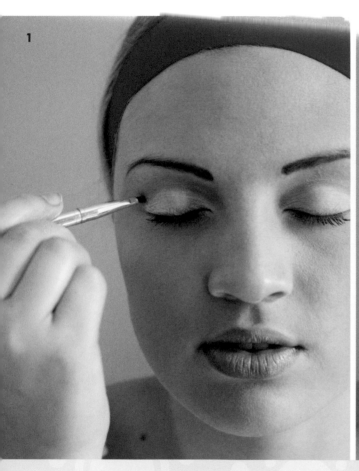

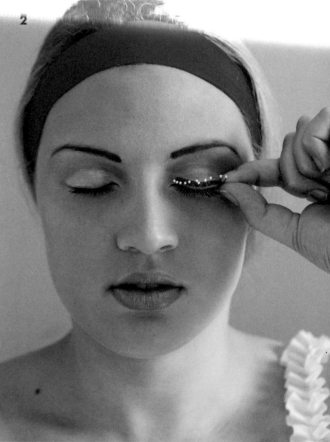

**1** Bold eyes need to be balanced by a strong brow to frame the face, so brush your eyebrows neatly into shape and define the arch using a brow pencil or powder. Then apply your eye-shadow(s) as desired. Here, a wash of white colour was brushed over the entire lid area to provide a smooth base. Then, using a small brush, the socket line was defined with blue eye-shadow. If you have very pale lashes, apply a coat of black mascara.

**2** Measure your false lashes by holding them up against your natural lash line. It is likely that the false lashes will be much longer, in which case, cut off the excess where the lashes are longest. Be cautious: trim a small amount off and measure again. Do this until the lashes are the correct length. Assuming the lashes are not pre-glued, manipulate each strip around your finger to create a soft curve that will help the lashes stick and sit flush against your eyelid.

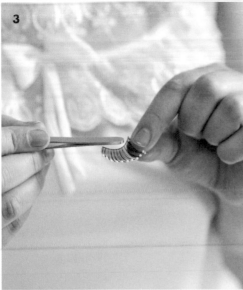

**3** Using the blunt end of a pair of tweezers, apply a film of lash glue to the false lashes, ensuring that you give it a few seconds to become 'tacky' before you position them on your lash line. I prefer using black lash glue, but you can also use the white lash glue that dries transparent.

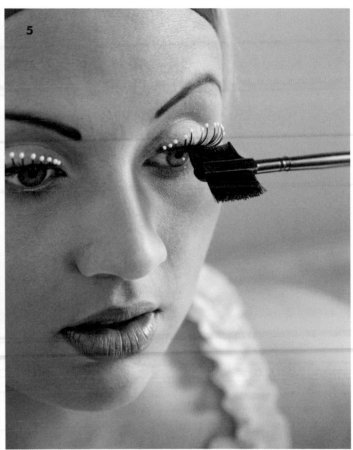

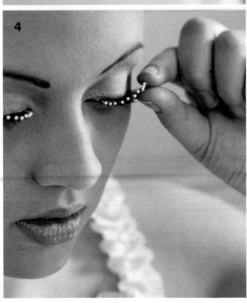

**4** Position the false lashes as close to your natural lash line as possible and manoeuvre them so they are flush against the skin. This may take some practice, so it is advisable to consider putting on your false lashes before any of your other make-up, including base, in case you make a mistake and need to remove them and clean off the lash glue. Once you have the application mastered, you can leave your lashes until later in the process. Squeeze them firmly in place between your thumb and forefinger all the way along.

**5** Using a lash comb, blend your natural and false lashes together. If you are wearing a particularly heavy or decorated style, you may not need to apply mascara; however, if you are wearing natural-style lashes, add mascara as desired.

# Beehive Yourself

*The beehive can be as vertiginous as you please, depending on the occasion and your mood. In the 1960s women often slept in their hives, wrapping them*

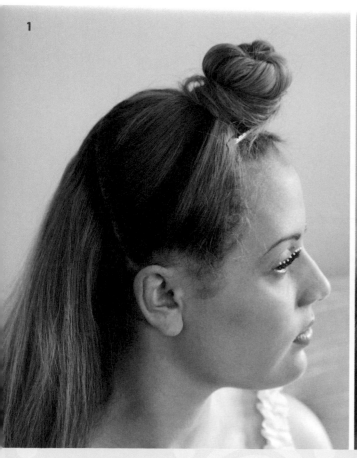

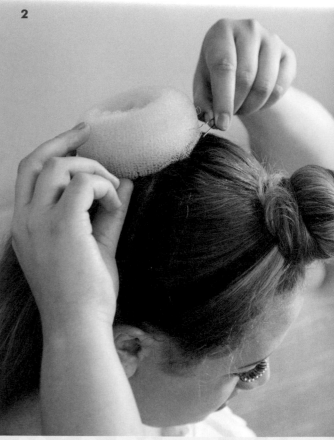

**1** Using the end of a pin-tail comb, divide your hair in half, separating the front from the back. Do this by taking a section across your head from your crown to the top of each ear, one side at a time. Try to keep your sectioning neat, as this will help you to achieve symmetry in your finished hairstyle. Brush the front section forward neatly and clip it on top of the front of your head.

**2** Place the hair donut centrally on the crown of your head, over the parting, and pin it in place all the way round to ensure it is held securely in position.

**3**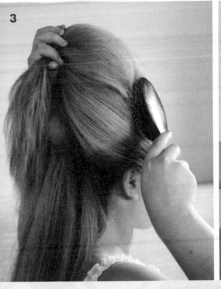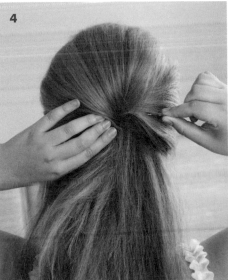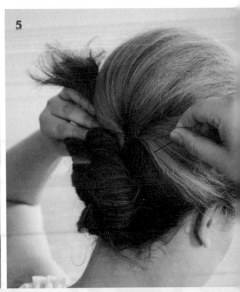

**3** Gently backcomb the front section of your hair from the roots to midway along its length. With the brush, lightly sweep the front section of your hair over the donut so it is covered. For a slightly softer look, leave out your fringe/bangs, if you have one, which you can style as desired – for instance, brush it to one side, pin it or curl it.

**4** Keeping the top smooth, neatly twist the front section of your hair under the donut and pin it securely in place.

**5** Gently backcomb the remainder of your hair and brush it upwards. Twist the section and secure it underneath the donut with pins.

**6** To complete the look, tuck the ends of your hair under and pin neatly in place with hair grips/bobby pins. Smooth down any stray hairs and spritz with hairspray.

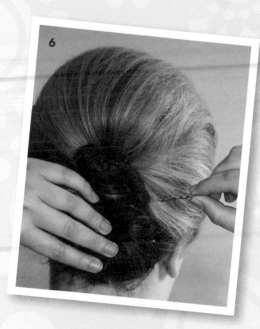

# Accessorizing This Look
## Groovy Baby

### accessories

Affordable 'plastic-fantastic' costume jewellery was churned out in abundance in the 1960s, often featuring chunky, bulbous beads and psychedelic or geometric patterns. Alice bands complemented beehives and it was also popular to tie a spare strip of fabric from a home-made or bespoke dress around the hair to match the outfit.

### fragrance

Popular fragrances tended to be overpowering and spicy, either leathery and masculine or ultra-sweet and feminine. Women seeking authentic vintage odours should check out Madame Rochas by Rochas (1960), with its pungent sandalwood, cedar and tonka bean, Yves Saint Laurent's Y (1964), with its lingering amber and oakmoss, or Guy Laroche's tropical Fidji (1966), which owes its scent to ingredients including lemon, bergamot and carnation.

### shoes

Although high heels remained popular during the 1960s, amongst the rapidly growing Modernist subculture the Continental influence dominated and girls found their mode of transport on a hot date would be by Lambretta. This required some forward thinking in the footwear department and created a craze for slip-on, low block-heel designs, which would look fabulous but were also practical. Shoes were fashioned in a wide variety of styles, including lace-up and slingback, as well as becoming desirable in PVC material. The 'Go-Go' boot is a classic example of PVC footwear, calf- or knee-length, often with a small platform and a cut-out feature on the side of the boot, à la André Courrèges; team with a bottom-scraping mini dress, if you dare.

> *Plastic, which was easy to colour, was the material of the moment.*

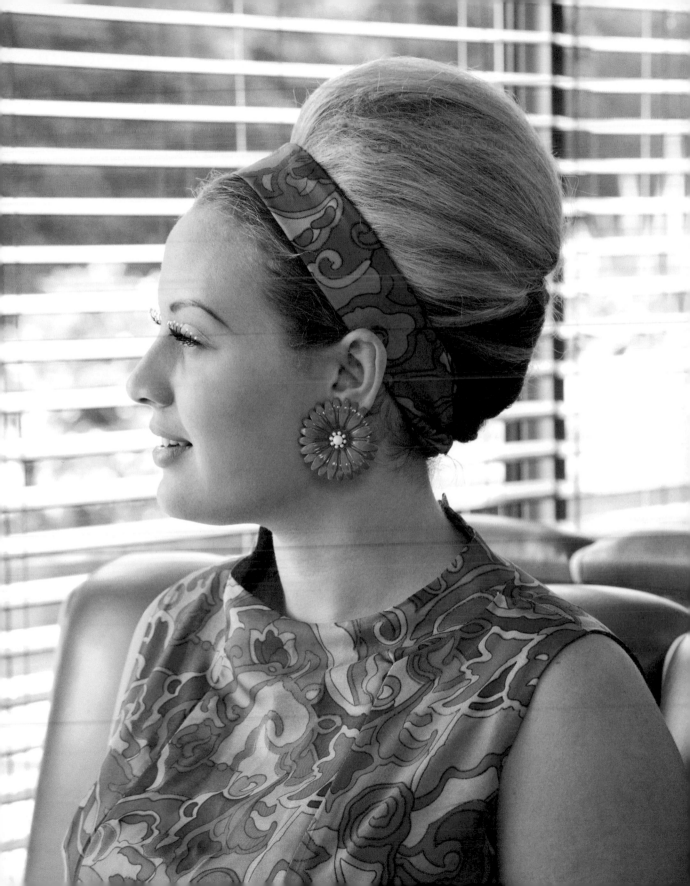

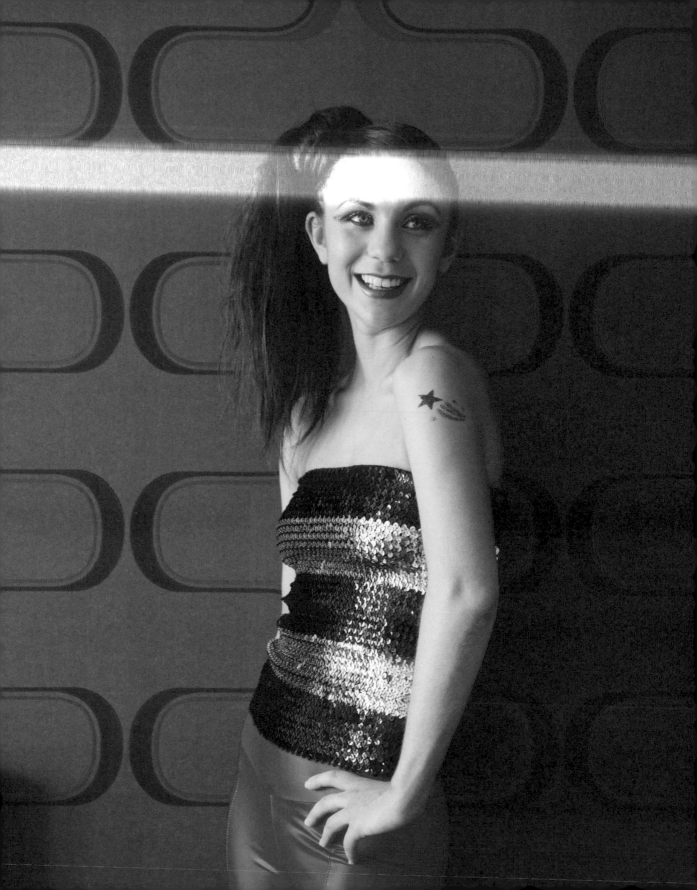

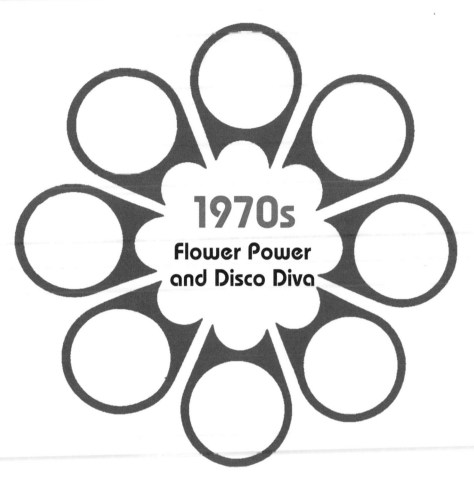

# 1970s
## Flower Power and Disco Diva

*The 'flower power' vibe of the late sixties continued into the first half of the 1970s, and the trademark long, flowing locks and barely there make-up of the hippies prevailed. As the decade progressed, a more glamorous look came to the fore, as Glam Rock and disco fever dominated the music scene: glitter, flicks and Afros were the last word.*

# The Free-spirited Seventies

The 1960s had become the era of free sexual liberation that was released through the backbone of teaching, and although the concept of free love was still coursing through the veins of many well into the 1970s, a reversal of modesty in design tantalized the mind rather than feasted the eyes. Orange and yellow were the dominating colours and according to the principles of colour therapy, orange relates to self-respect and yellow to self-worth. With political unrest in both the UK and the USA, perhaps the governments of the day were surreptitiously experimenting with ways to manipulate the mind of individuals on the cusp of a revolt against the three-day week, decimalization and the Vietnam War. From a fashion perspective, the decade was simply blindingly bright.

Hair and make-up lurched between the two ends of the spectrum. Individuals could chose a 'natural' look, favouring centre-parted, tousled styles, which embraced all hair textures, and minimal make-up. This largely fell under the category of 'hippie' and was a simple and low-maintenance approach to female grooming.

It wasn't until Farrah Fawcett-Majors burst onto the TV screens, along with Kate Jackson and Jaclyn Smith in 1976, that women reached for the rollers and styling irons once more. *Charlie's Angels* were revered by men and women alike.

At the other end of the scale, hair trends factored in the increasing tolerance of a multicultural society – while ignorance and racism still prevailed, fashion attempted inclusivity. Afro-perms became all the rage, especially on the mid-decade disco scene. At the same time, Ziggy Stardust and Glam Rock were seemingly responsible for fathers giving their sons 'a good talking to', as the theatrical, bi-curious music master became an instant success, sporting a lurex cat suit, towering platforms, dyed hair and brightly coloured makeup.

By the last years of the decade, Malcolm McLaren and Vivienne Westwood were the King and Queen of Punk, holding court at their shop on London's King's Road. The movement was epitomized by the controversial statement looks involving extreme clothing, dramatic make-up, shaved heads and Mohawk hairstyles.

*make-up colour palette:*

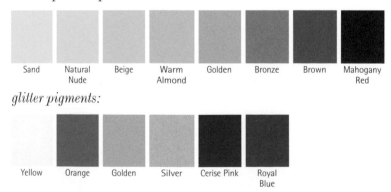

| Sand | Natural Nude | Beige | Warm Almond | Golden | Bronze | Brown | Mahogany Red |

*glitter pigments:*

| Yellow | Orange | Golden | Silver | Cerise Pink | Royal Blue |

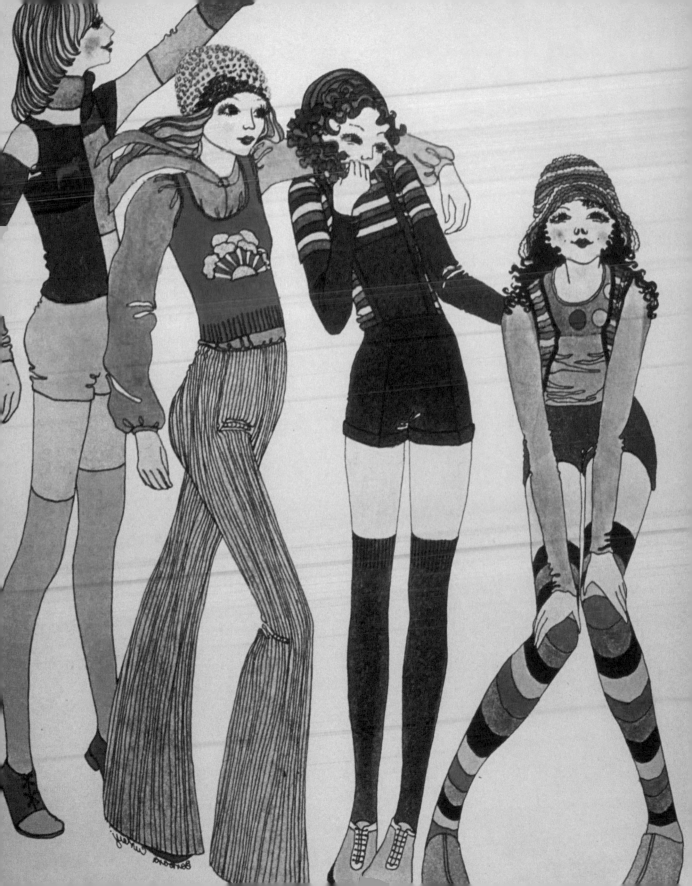

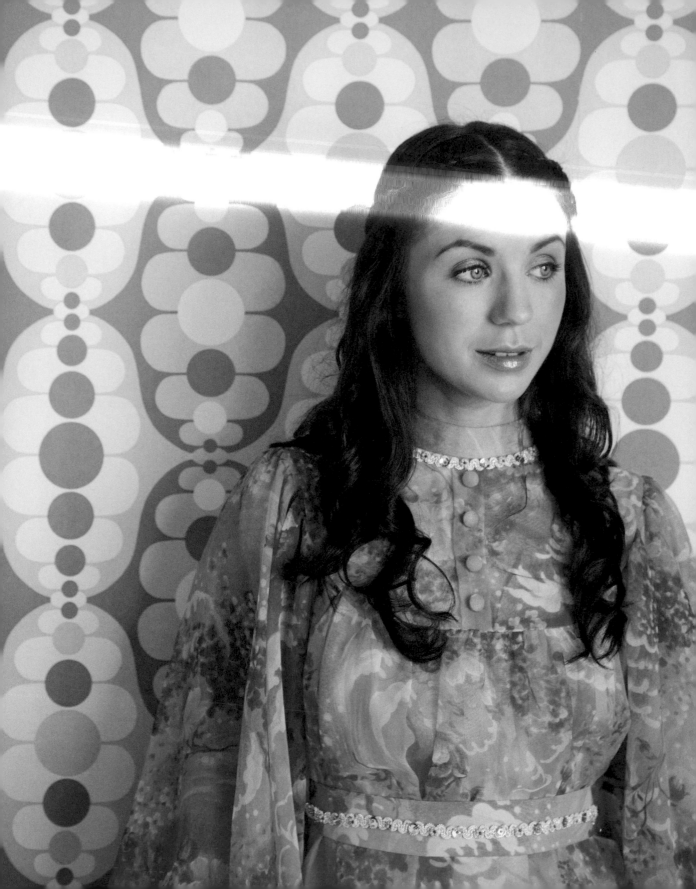

# Flower Power

*This relaxed look can work with leisurely daytime attire or for the hostess with the mostest re-creating her very own 'Abigail's Party'. The laid-back, low-maintenance mood also makes it perfect for festivals.*

During the 1970s the cosmetics world experienced ever-growing product development and, in particular, saw the rise in demand for sunless tanning products following reports in the media of the link between excessive UV exposure and the development of certain carcinomas. Bronzers helped women achieve a radiant glow and were typically worn with layered mascara and clear lip gloss to accentuate their natural beauty.

When re-creating this look, those with porcelain skin should avoid dark bronzers and instead try a gradual sunless tanner, which can be applied over the course of a few days to build up a colour appropriate for your skin tone. For evening, add an eye-shadow of your choice with a soft-pearl finish and deepen the colour of your lips using a natural 'bitten lip' stain topped with slick of gloss. Most shimmery bronzers contain mica, which gives a glistening effect, but you can easily find matte bronzers that work well for shading, too.

Hair should ideally be left free from styling products; however, a small amount of serum or shine spray will give your locks a healthy lustre.

## TO CREATE THIS LOOK YOU WILL NEED:

### MAKE-UP
Liquid bronzer in a shade suitable for your skin tone * black or dark brown eyeliner pencil * medium eye-shadow brush * taupe-grey pearlized eye-shadow * lip stain * clear lip gloss

### HAIR
Hairbrush * pin-tail or medium-tooth comb * sectioning clips * bendy rollers and a hairdryer or set of heated rollers * hair grips/bobby pins * hairspray

# Beautiful Bronze

*To create a natural glow, choose a bronzer that is only a shade or two deeper*
*than your natural skin tone and build up the colour gradually, concentrating*
*on the parts of your face that naturally catch the sun.*

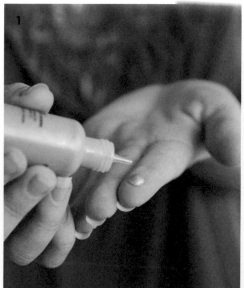

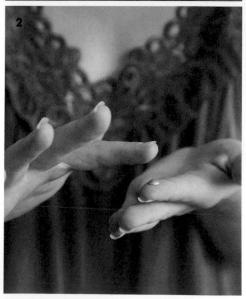

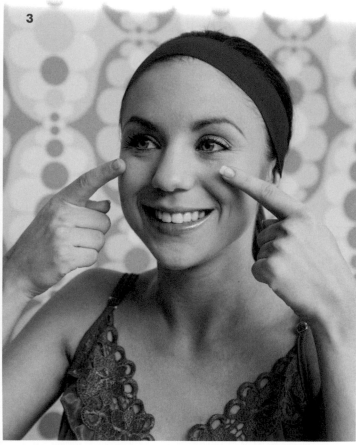

**1** Making sure your hands are clean and dry, apply a pea-size amount of liquid bronzer to the tip of your index finger.

**2** Gently dab the liquid onto the index finger of the other hand, as this will prevent you from applying too much product and will allow you to create an even distribution of bronzer on your face.

**3** Using small, circular motions, apply the bronzer to your cheek area only, working from the highest point of the 'apples' in an upwards and outwards motion towards your temples. Take care to blend it well and make sure that it doesn't settle into any fine lines.

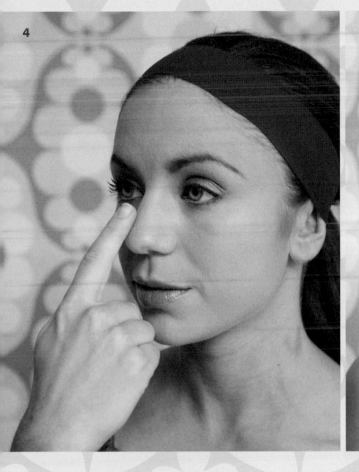

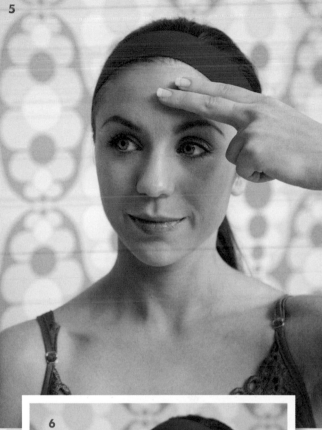

**4** Using the index finger of one hand, apply a light coat of bronzer to the bridge of your nose in a sweeping motion, blending it well, as before.

**5** Using the index and middle finger of the other hand, apply a light coat of bronzer across your forehead in a sweeping motion. Blend it carefully to ensure that it doesn't settle in any creases, and soften any hard edges.

**6** Lastly, apply a small dab of bronzer to your chin in a circular motion, using the index and middle fingers of both hands. This method of application will limit the bronzer to the areas that would naturally be 'kissed' by the sun and gives your make-up the most natural finish.

# Soft Waves

*Bendy rollers, which you can heat up using a hairdryer, work best for irregular, loose waves, but standard heated rollers can also be used. If your hair doesn't curl easily, you may find that using a styling product helps.*

**1** Brush your hair to remove the knots and smooth out tangles. Create a middle parting using a pin-tail or medium tooth comb. Then, make a section on either side of your parting at the front, about 5 cm/2 inches above your ears and stopping about 5 cm/2 inches away from your hairline. Twist these sections individually and pin them out of the way on the top of your head with sectioning clips while you set the rest of your hair in the rollers.

**2** Roll up the back sections of the hair, starting at the nape and working up. The hair is not being set right up to the roots, so leave out the roots, concentrating on the lengths of the hair, so that the resulting waves will lie close to the head. If the rollers you are using vary in size, use the larger ones on the top sections, scaling down to the smaller size at the base of the neck. Heat up the rollers using a hairdryer, if necessary, and then allow to set.

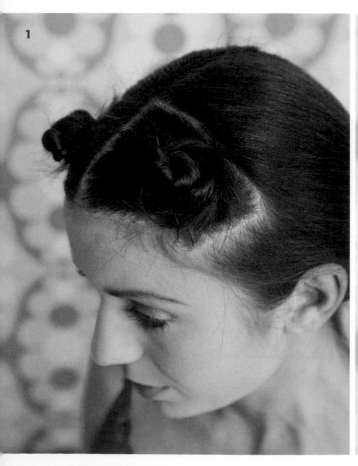

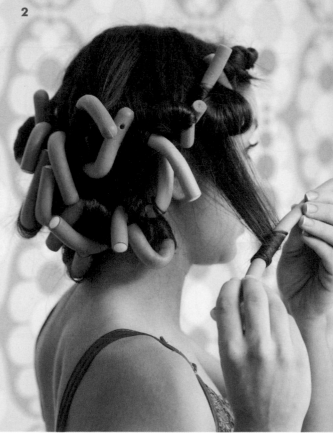

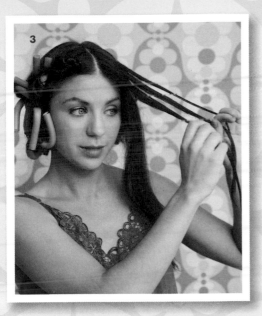

**3** Ensure you leave the rollers in until the hair is completely cool to allow the curls to fix in shape, then remove them and separate the curls gently with your fingers. Unpin the front section and take a small section at the front of it and divide that into three smaller sections. You can do this with your fingers or with the pin-tail comb.

**4** Begin making a plait, adding in small sections of hair evenly from the hairline as you work. Continue plaiting through to the ends.

**5** Secure the finished plait with grips/bobby pins at the back of the head. Repeat on the other side and blast with hairspray to finish.

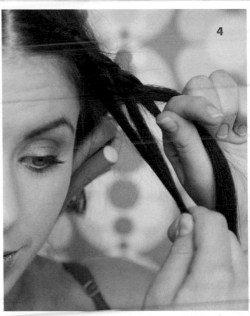

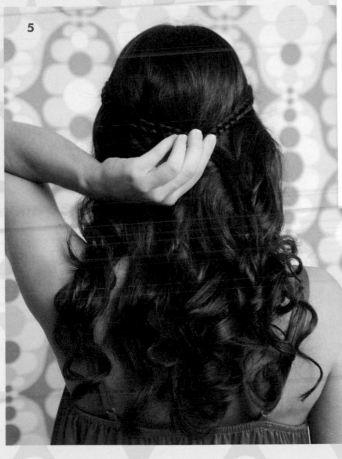

# Accessorizing This Look
## Flower Power

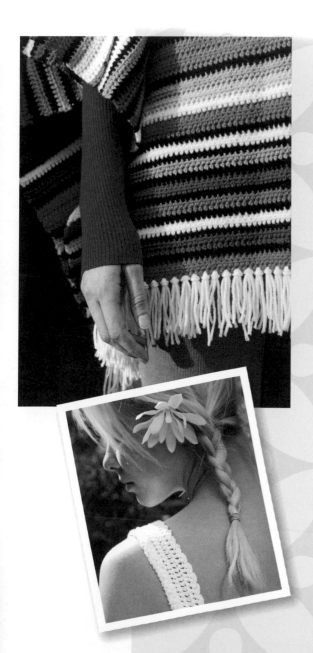

### crochet

Used in almost
every element
of fashion – from
hair clips and bags
to cardigans and stockings – crochet was taken to a whole
new level in the 1970s. Items crocheted with natural thick
fibres along with man-made synthetic materials tend to
have stood the test of time, so look out for these when
shopping for original retro pieces. Alternatively, invest in
some crochet hooks and get creative. This skill, along with
knitting, has seen a revival and, with a bit of basic
training, the options are limitless.

### flowers

Wearing real flowers symbolized a connection with nature
and they were often used as hair accessories, bracelets or
necklaces – think daisy chain on a summer's day. However,
synthetic flowers – such as daisies, buttercups or exotic
blooms in yellow, orange or cerise – can be added to hair,
clothes and bags for an authentic flower power vibe.

### hats

Although hats as everyday wear lost a battle with
popularity in the mid-1960s, floppy wide-brimmed hats
were all the rage in the 1970s. Summer versions look great
worn with a kaftan, while heavier material, such as felt,
will add a touch of boho chic to a winter outfit.

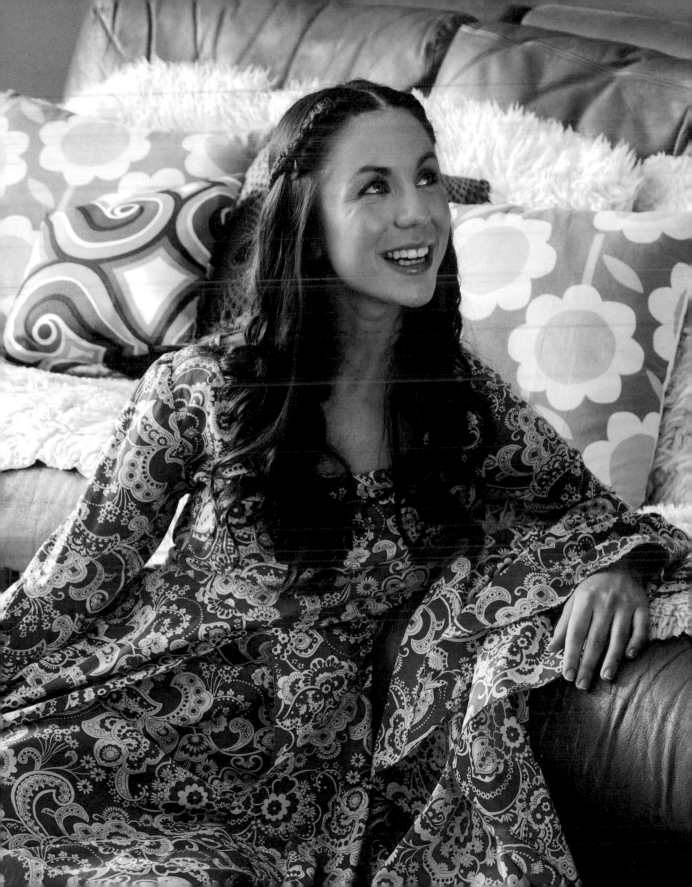

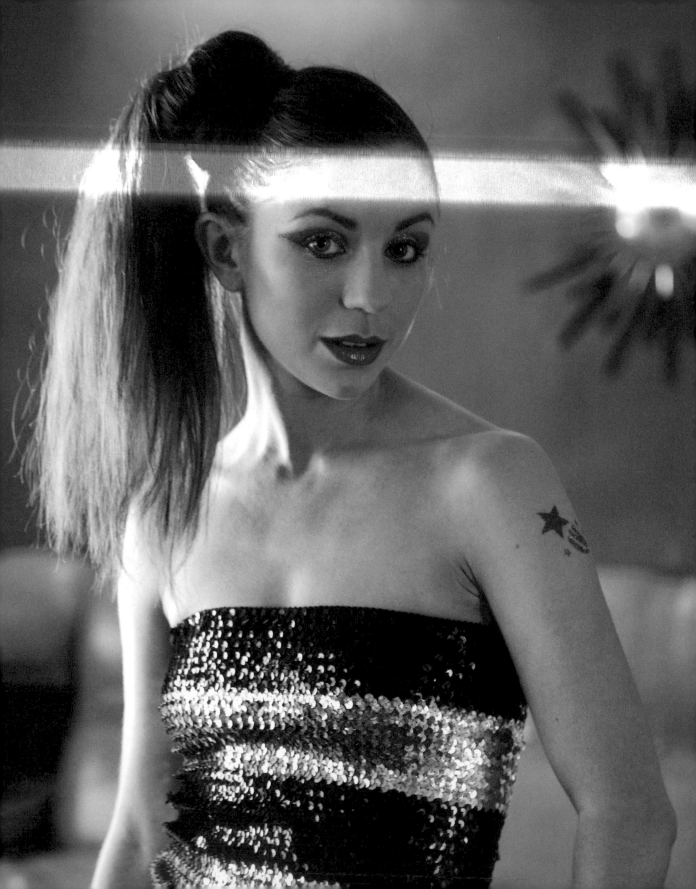

# Disco Diva

*Perfect for parties, this side-swept pony allows the hair to retain an element of movement but keeps it off the face, which is not only practical when dancing, but also elongates the neck and shows off the bold make-up.*

Compelling for its colourful costumes, psychedelic lighting and irresistible groove that encouraged freedom of expression, disco soon had a far wider following than the African American and Latino club-goers of New York and Philadelphia where it originated. Mainstream on both sides of the Atlantic for most of the decade, disco was dramatic, and hairstyles needed to be able to withstand high-impact dance-floor gyrations. Make-up, too, needed staying power, and shimmery textures and bold colours struck the right note on dance floors everywhere. Glitter and face paint, along with liquid eye-shadow, featured prominently on the cosmetics shelves in the seventies, and although it was more geared towards the youthful market, it was bought by the masses.

Cosmetics containing mica catch the light and work exceptionally well to create a shimmering effect that accentuates the area of application. Worn with a subtle hint of bronzer and lashings of lip gloss, you will look like a regular at The Loft – a member's-only dance club set up by DJ David Mancuso in New York in 1970 and one of the first discos.

## TO CREATE THIS LOOK YOU WILL NEED:

### MAKE-UP
Mixing-medium gel ✳ white eye glitter ✳ eye-shadow brush ✳ deep pink glitter eye-shadow ✳ eyeliner brush ✳ pink glitter gel eyeliner ✳ glitter mascara

### HAIR
Bristle hairbrush ✳ hair band ✳ hair donut ✳ hair grips/bobby pins ✳ pin-tail comb ✳ hairspray

# Glam Glitter

*Glitter is messy to apply, so it is a good idea to do your eyes before the rest of your make-up. Cat's-eye flicks usually require very precise application, but shimmery textures are much more forgiving of mistakes than flat colours.*

1 Dab a little shiny cream base over your eyelids with the pad of your finger, concentrating on the eyelid, socket and brow bone. Clean and dry your finger immediately to prevent smearing the gel anywhere else. If you prefer, you can use a cotton bud/Q-tip or eye-shadow brush to apply the gel.

2 Dip the index finger of your other hand into the white eye glitter and dab this over your eyelids, really pressing the gel, focusing on the inner half of the eye. Build up the intensity as desired and make sure that you have an even distribution of glitter on both eyelids. Once again, you can use a cotton bud/Q-tip or an eye shadow brush to do this if you prefer.

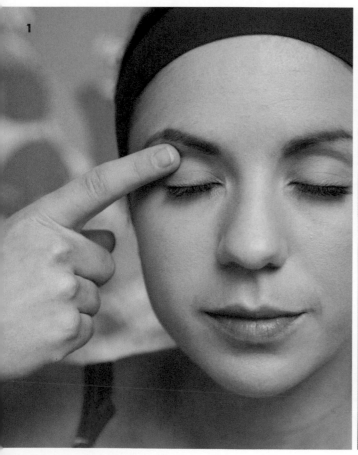

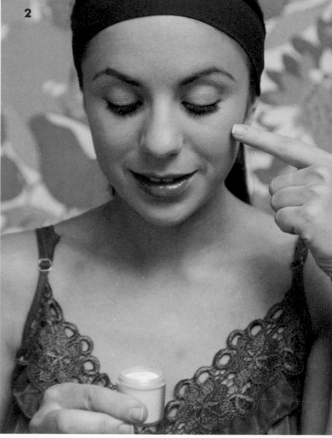

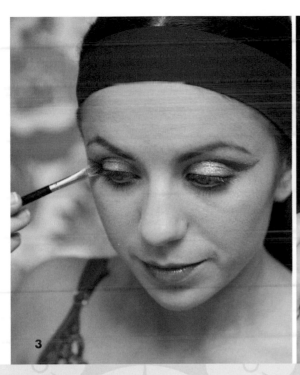

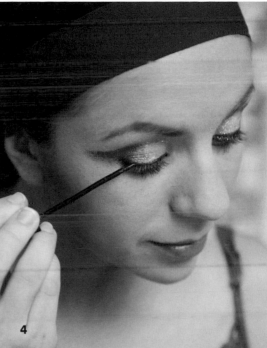

**3** Using an eye-shadow brush rather than your finger for greater precision, apply deep pink glitter eye-shadow along the socket crease, starting at the inner corner of the eye and taking it to the outer corner. Working carefully, take the colour horizontally beyond the outer corner of the eye to form a cat's-eye flick, and blend the colour onto the outer corner of the eye, taking it down the lid to the lash line at the outer corner only.

**4** With an eyeliner brush and a steady hand, apply deep pink glitter gel eyeliner along your upper and lower lash lines, working from the inner corners to the outer corners. As before, build up the intensity of colour as desired.

**5** Finish by applying three coats of glitter mascara to your top and bottom lashes, allowing each coat to dry before you apply the next.

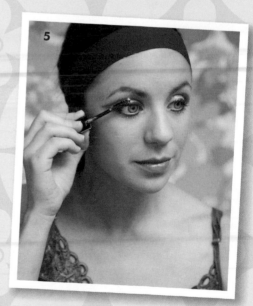

# Side Ponytail

*This versatile look will see you onto the dance floor and beyond. You can make it as dramatic as you please, with extra height and volume, or opt for a sleek, sophisticated version that wouldn't look out of place with your LBD.*

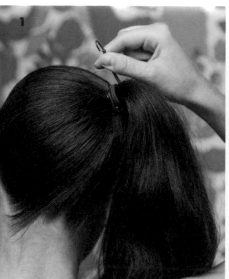 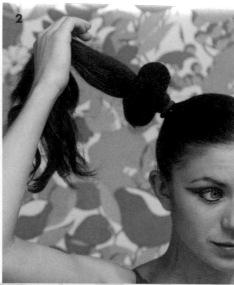 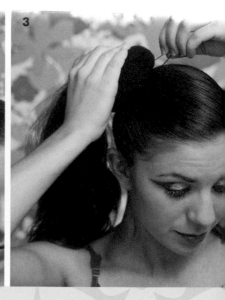

**1** Take all your hair and, using a bristle brush, sweep it over to one side and gather it into a ponytail approximately 5 cm/2 inches above your ear. Adjust the height of your ponytail according to the length of your hair – make it lower for shorter hair and higher for longer hair. When you are happy with the position of the side ponytail, secure it with a hair band.

**2** Pull your ponytail through a hair donut. If necessary, smooth any stray strands of frizzy hair with a spritz of shine spray before pulling it though.

**3** Secure the donut with hair grips/bobby pins. Keep in mind that if you intend to do some high-energy dancing, the donut could slip, so make sure that you use enough hair grips/bobby pins to hold it securely in place.

*Positioning the ponytail at the side is what gives it the 1970s vibe.*

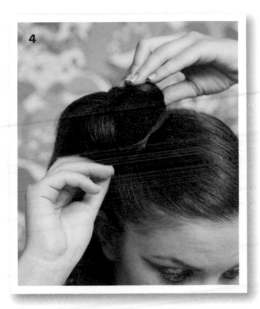

**4** Take individual sections of your hair and place them around the donut to cover it. You can be as creative in the way you wrap the strands around the donut as you like. Secure the hair with hair grips/bobby pins as you work.

**5** Try to take sections of hair evenly from all round the donut, working from the top in one direction all the way around and leaving the middle section as a loose ponytail inside the 'knot'.

**6** Once the donut is completely covered and the 'knot' secured with plenty of hair grips/bobby pins, lightly backcomb the remaining ponytail to give it extra volume. Tease it into shape with the end of your pin-tail comb and smooth down any stray hairs around your face. Finally, spritz the hair with hairspray to hold it in place.

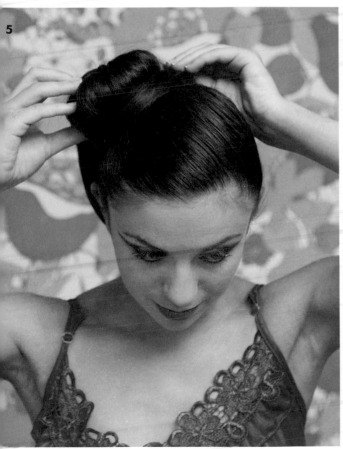

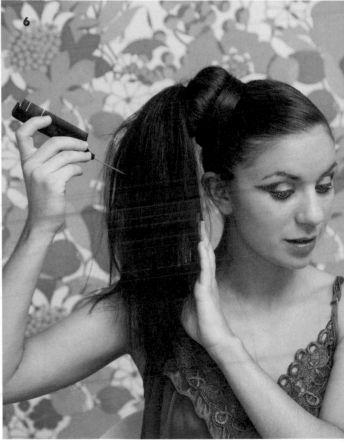

# Accessorizing This Look
## Disco Diva

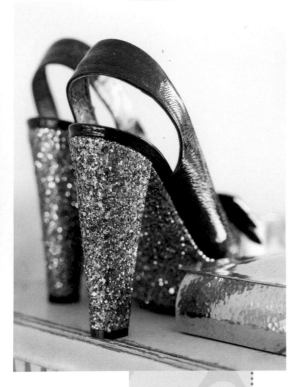

### fragrance

An established cosmetics house since the 1930s, Revlon developed a new fragrance for women in 1973. Charlie was an instant hit, and in a bid to rival Estée by Estée Lauder, Revlon launched Charlie Blue later the same year. The advertising campaign controversially featured the first African American woman ever to be used in a cosmetics campaign. Both fragrances have stood the test of time and are readily available today.

### glitter & sequins

From headbands to boob tubes, almost every item of eveningwear sparkled, glistened and reflected in the disco ball. Many modern designers have sought inspiration from the days of disco – Christian Louboutin recently gave the world of footwear a glitter-fest with the Pigale Mini Glitter Pumps, as did Stella McCartney. If your budget stretches to designer, indulge; if not, second-hand shops, charity shops and retro stores tend to provide rich pickings.

### shoes

Platforms dominated the decade. From modest 2.5-cm/1-inch sandals to skyscraping 10-cm/5-inch-plus knee-high boots, it was all about height – slingbacks being the most precarious options. Despite the widely held belief that retro shopping is a relatively modern trend, it was the 1970s that saw second-hand shopping become fashionable. Wearing pre-loved items had been considered a shameful necessity by those living in poverty, but midway through the decade, thrifty fashionistas wore yesteryear's garments as a statement. Styles of the 1930s and 1940s experienced a huge revival, with some delicate twists, so consider art-deco-style dance shoes and high-heeled brogues as part of your seventies wardrobe.

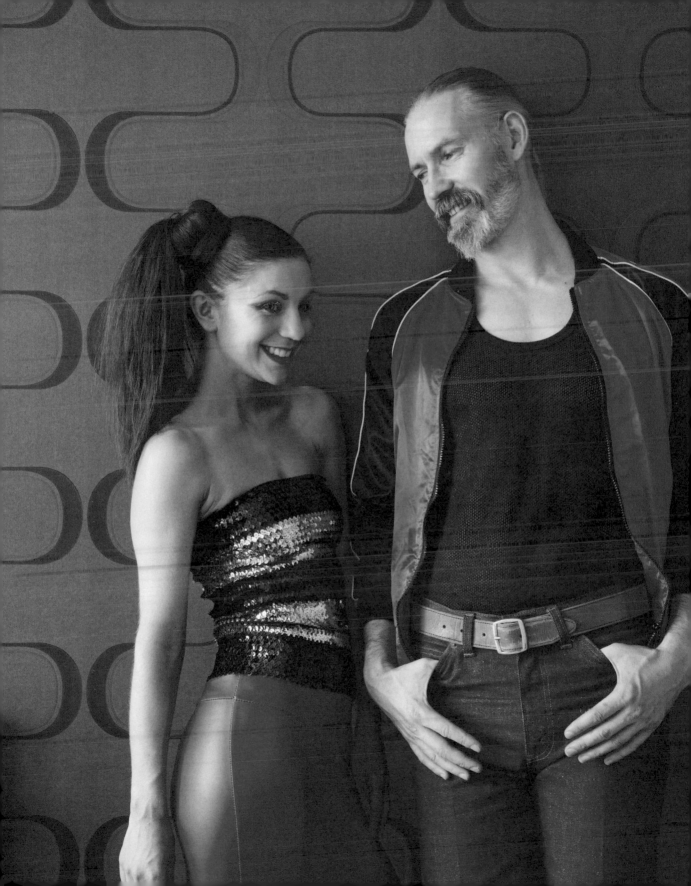

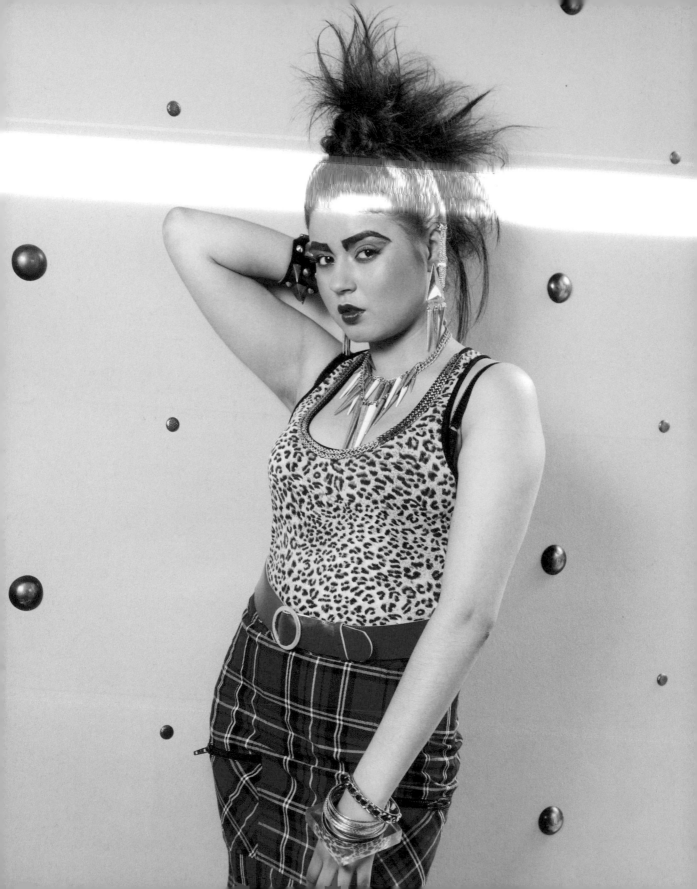

# 1980s
## Safety Pin-Up and Punk-Tuition

*Often dubbed the decade that fashion forgot, the 1980s
gave us everything from Punks and New Romantics to
power dressing and dancewear. Michael Jackson and
Madonna were the King and Queen of Pop, Dallas and
Dynasty dominated the TV screens and Princess Diana
graced the covers of magazines around the world.*

# The Flamboyant Eighties

By the time the seventies edged to a close, the variation in subcultures had widened to such an extent that fashion for hair and make-up styles was continually altering at a warp speed. Punks, Goths, Yuppies, New Romantics, Preppies – the list was endless and the mindset was 'anything goes.'

As the new decade dawned, resistance to radical social and economic change was given an elevated platform on the catwalks of the world as fashion got political. Awareness of worldwide suffering was no more apparent than when 2 billion people in 60 countries tuned in to watch *Live Aid* in 1985. The human race had recoiled in horror two years previously at the discovery, by doctors at the Pasteur Institute in France, of AIDS, a new and incurable disease that threatened millions of people worldwide. The Cold War and the Iran-Iraq War monopolized headlines, and in 1989 walls were literally broken down to unite Eastern Europe once more.

Product development went into overdrive in the 1980s and the hair and cosmetics industry found itself besieged with brands, all vying for consumer attention. Curls were united with a new product called mousse, and hair art became constructional with the development of sculpting gels and hairsprays, enabling some styles to resemble edifices. Even 'everyday' hair

became enormous, as women scrunched and teased their locks upwards and outwards. Hair dye also reached a peak in sales, as blonde highlights as well as less conventional colour streaks were requested. Then there was crimping. Crimpers were, without fail, the decade's favourite hair tool. Contemporary crimpers were invented by Geri Cucenza in the early 1970s, but it wasn't until the following decade that they ended up on every girl's wish list.

To complement the big hair, shoulder pads and oversized tops, often worn over leggings, a ra-ra skirt or skin-tight acid-washed jeans, make-up was bold and bright. Sharp-angled eyebrows framed strong-coloured eyes, teamed with bright neon or frosted-pink lips and bold blusher. Tattoos and piercings found a new, broader audience in Western society. Celebrity androgyny and pansexuality sparked a craze for make-up and hairstyles to be shared by both sexes. Revellers at London nightclubs such as Taboo, Blitz and Kinky Gerlinky were particularly noted for their unique creativity and outrageous flamboyance. Those seeking a less theatrical appearance sought influence from pop stars, notably Madonna and Cindy Lauper. Actresses and supermodels also provided inspiration, with Brooke Shields championing the natural bushy eyebrow and Cindy Crawford becoming almost solely responsible for the drawn-on mole.

*make-up colour palette:*

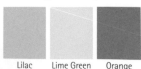    

Lilac | Lime Green | Orange | Cerise Pink | Silver | Black

*frosted colours:*

  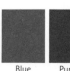

White | Yellow | Golden | Cherry Red | Blue | Purple

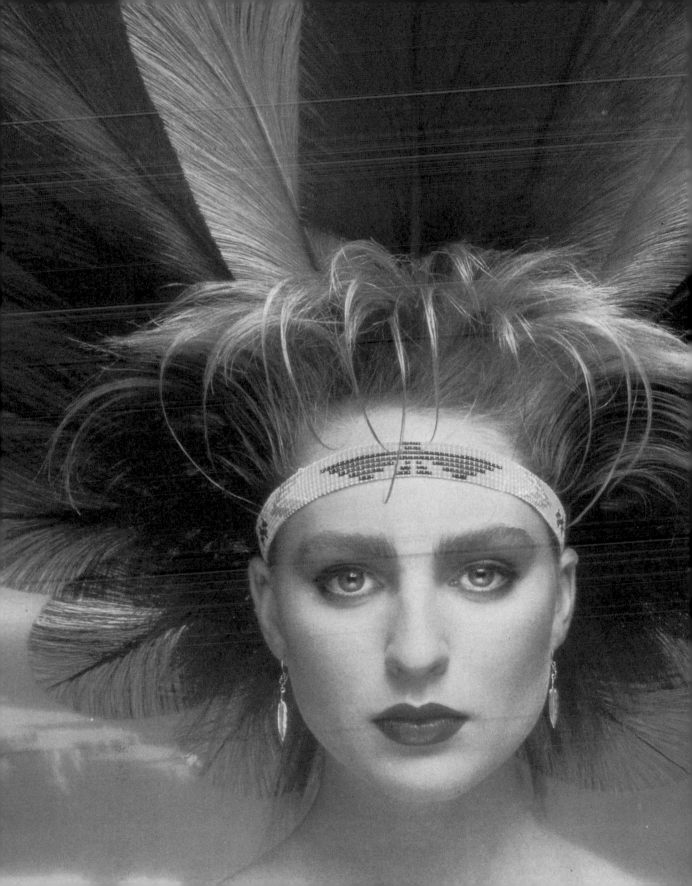

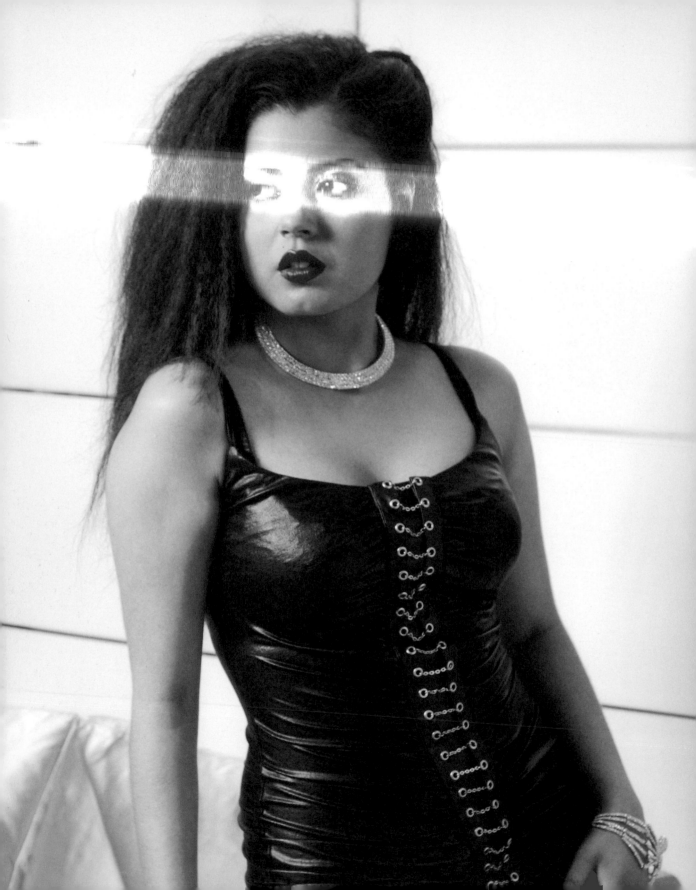

# Safety Pin-Up

*This sexy party look is a crossbreed of Dynasty-inspired glamour, New Romantica and the Goth subculture. The versatile smoky eye is given a distinct eighties flavour by pairing it with bold, bright lips and big, crimped hair.*

This look celebrates some of the keynotes of the decade, when bone-crushing body-con was frequently offset by frills and ruffles, and accessorized with safety pins, chokers and strappy shoes with razor-sharp points. Raven-black hair is teased upwards and outwards, while eyes and lips are accentuated with heavy, dark, shimmery make-up. Peppered with a hint of sado-masochistic erotica, this is a statement looks that needs to be worn with attitude.

While this interpretation would be perfect for a vampiric Halloween party, the smoky eye doesn't have to be shades of grey, and you can also get creative with spray-on, wash-out hair colour. This became hugely popular in the 1980s, when, much as with piercings and tattoos, radically changing the colour of the hair, even on a semi-permanent basis, was too much of a commitment for some. There are an abundance of colours to choose from and, if you are feeling particularly adventurous, you could consider using two or three colours on the roots and ends for maximum impact.

## To create this look you will need:

### Make-up
Small eye-shadow brush * white eye-shadow * metallic silver eye-shadow * medium, flat, round-edged eye-shadow brush * metallic black eye-shadow * black kohl eyeliner pencil * black mascara * lash and brow comb * brow pencil or powder * red lipstick

### Hair
Crimping irons * natural-bristle hairbrush * medium-tooth comb * hair grips/bobby pins * wash-out colour spray * hairspray

# Smoky Eyes

*The smoky eye is a classic evening look that can be made more or less dramatic, as you wish, simply by adding more layers of the deepest colour.*

*The easy to do this look . . . the secret is to blend the colours really well.*

**1** Using a . . . eye shadow brush, apply . . . shadow at the innermost corner of your socket, taking it over the eyelid and up to the socket crease. This gives a brightening effect and makes your eyes look bigger. Blend it softly into the crease to soften the edges.

**2** Take take . . . the silver eye shadow and apply as a continuation . . . to the socket your socket, starting about a third of the way in from the corner of the eye and taking it right to the outer corner. Blend the colours well, so that they merge seemlessly without an obvious line.

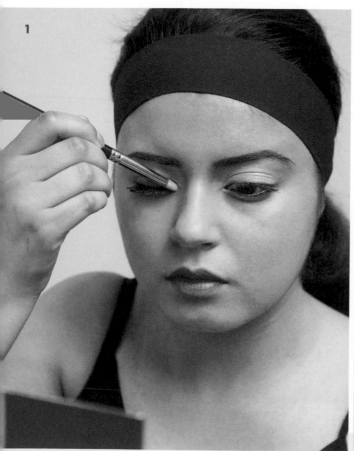

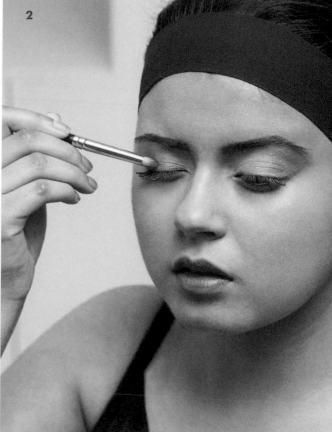

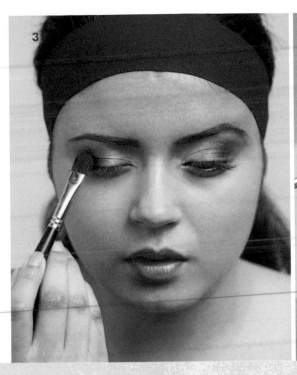

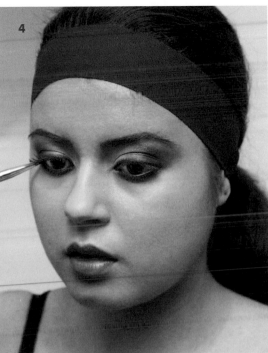

**3** Using a flat, round-edged eye-shadow brush, apply metallic black eye-shadow to the outer third of the eye and into the socket crease to create depth. Sweep it outwards and upwards to create a 'cat's-eye' effect. Use the edge of the brush to work the colour into the crease and define the shape around the eye socket. A little goes a long way, so add the colour gradually, building it up to the desired intensity.

**4** With the edge of the same brush, apply a line of metallic black eye-shadow along the outer part of the lower lash line and smudge it to create a smoky effect.

**5** Line the inner part of the lower lash line with a soft black kohl pencil and coat the lashes with lots of black mascara.

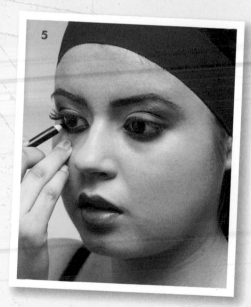

# 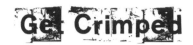Get Crimped

*Whether you had a mullet, a rat tail or a long asymmetric fringe/bangs, or a*
*predilection for scrunchies or headbands, crimping your mane was de rigueur*
*in the eighties and crimping irons were an vital piece of kit for men and women.*

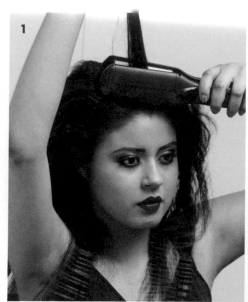

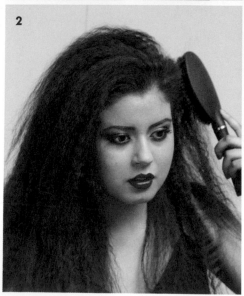

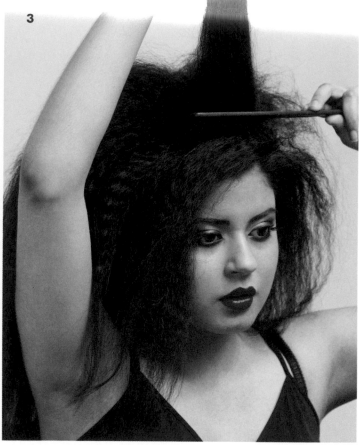

**1** Apply heat-protection spray before you start, if you wish, and work on dry hair. Take a section of hair approximately 4 cm/1½ inches in width. Starting at the roots, place the hair inside the crimping irons and hold for ten seconds, then release. Reposition the crimpers farther down the same length of hair and repeat, working your way down to the ends. Repeat this process until all of your hair is crimped.

**2** Brush the hair through with a natural-bristle hairbrush.

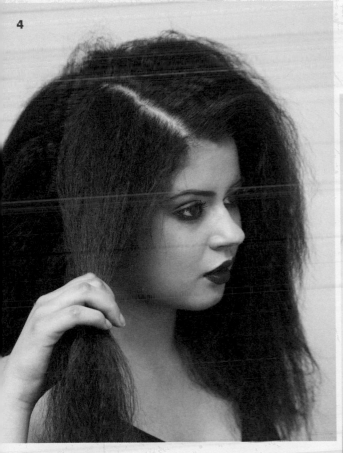

**4**

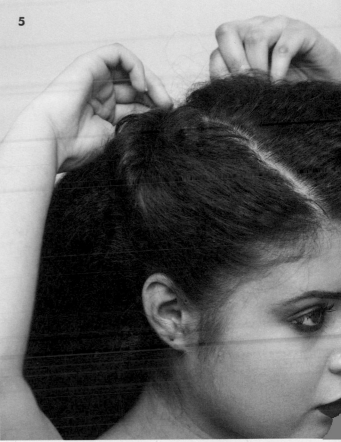

**5**

**3** To create extra volume, backcomb the hair in sections, using a comb. Focus on the underneath areas to give additional lift at the roots and smooth down the top.

**4** Take a section of hair at one side of the head, from the hairline to the top of the ear.

**5** Twist that section of hair away from your face a few times and secure it at the crown of your head with a couple of hair grips/bobby pins.

If you wish, spray the ends of your hair with a wash-out colour of your choice, and spritz with hairspray to hold.

# Accessorizing This Look
## Safety Pin-Up

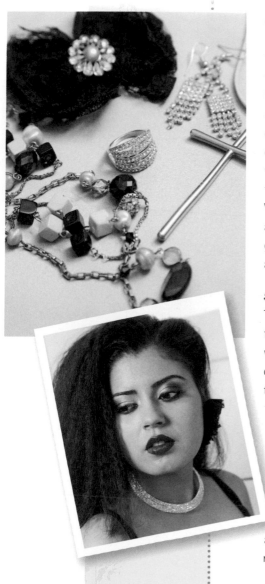

### costume jewellery

Costume jewellery was available in every price range. Often fashioned from inexpensive plastics and metals, many items at the time contained nickel, to which many people are allergic, so be wary when purchasing vintage pieces as reactions can be quite uncomfortable. Hoop earrings, chain-linked studs and enormous diamonté clip-on earrings were all in demand – as with many other things in the 1980s, it was a case of 'the bigger, the better' when it came to earrings. Multiple bangles and crucifixes were also fashionable. At the other end of the scale, designers such as Dior, Versace and Chanel were offering chunky statement pieces that are highly collectable today, including brooches and chain belts. A good tip is to look out for named pieces of costume jewellery from any era, as this will most often signify quality as well as desirability.

### shoes

The footwear of the 1980s was influenced by a mishmash of styles from preceding decades. Everything from jellies to Doc Martens were in, but the ultimate powering-dressing female footwear of choice was undoubtedly the court shoe. The rounded-off-point-toe court shoe was a hybrid of the shapes popularized in the 1940s and 1950s and came in countless patterns. Pinet, Roland Cartier, Joan & David, Charles Jourdan and Gina – not forgetting Clarks – showcased collection upon collection of designs that can easily be found in vintage outlets and thrift stores worldwide. For those looking for something slightly edgier, search for creations with spiky stiletto heels, straps, buckles and laces, which will often bind the ankles and legs. Such designs were a fusion of Punk and erotica, which experimented with unusual materials in both footwear and clothing.

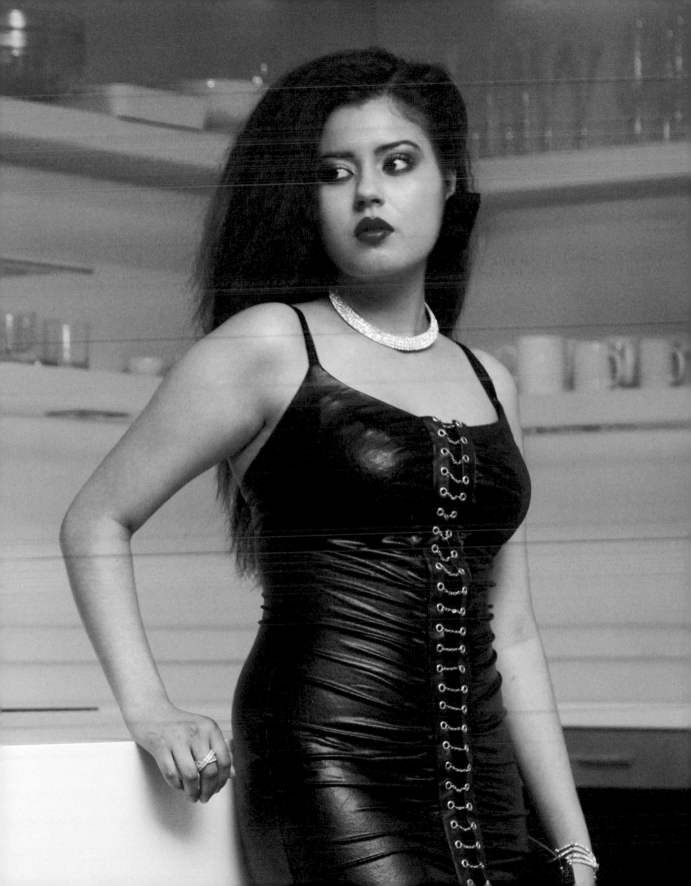

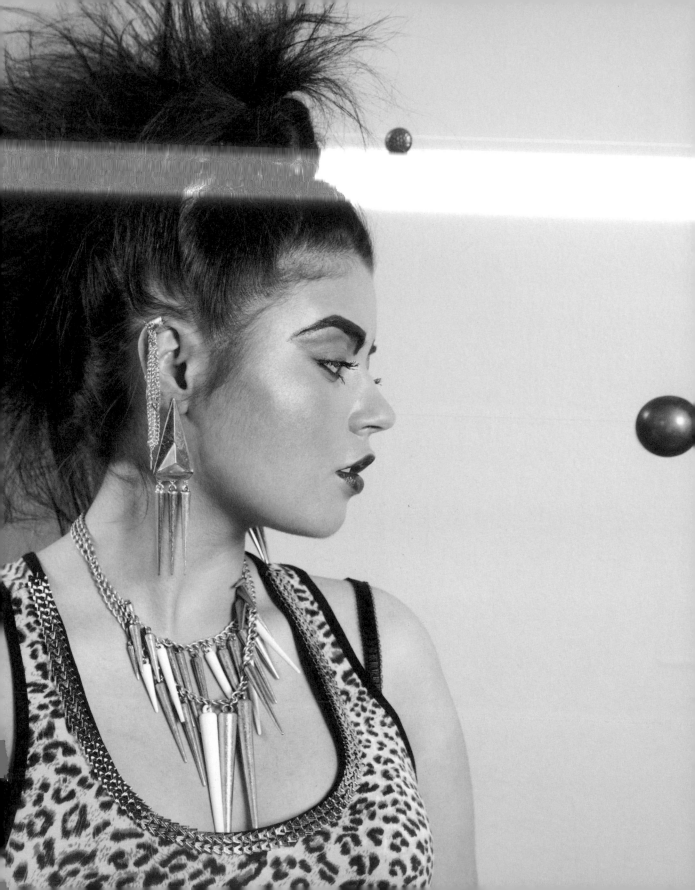

# Punk-Tuition

*Subversive, provocative and extreme, Punk fashion was designed to shock and make a statement. Anything goes, so be bold, have fun and experiment with bright coloured make-up and don't skimp on mousse, gel or hairspray.*

The 1980s were all about wearing bold colours and statement make-up, so don't be afraid to think 'outside the box' and create your own unique style. When you are designing make-up looks that will alter the shape of facial features, such as eyebrows and lips, it can be helpful to doodle your ideas on paper first, to see if your colour choices work. Then set aside some time to practise the finished look on your face.

Punk hairstyles were loud and proud. Hair was often bleached or dyed jet black or unnatural colours – bright pink, blue, orange, yellow, green, red or a rainbow combination of hues – and then fashioned into tall Mohawks or sculpted into spikes. The raft of modern styling products available today make it easy to re-create the Punk look without committing to a radical cut or colour change.

Theatre and art went hand in hand in the 1980s, so put on your ripped fishnets, tartan mini, studded jacket and bovver boots, and be prepared to strike a pose in the moshpit.

## To create this look you will need:

### Make-up
Medium fluff eye-shadow brush * light mauve eye-shadow * flat, angled eye-shadow brush * purple eye-shadow * rich blue eye-shadow * square-edged eyeliner brush * black or dark brown kohl pencil * bold blue pencil or liquid eyeliner * black mascara

### Hair
Natural-bristle hairbrush * medium-tooth comb * hair bands * hairspray * straightening irons * hair grips/bobby pins * wash-out colour spray

# Bold-Colour Eyes

*Bright colour-block designs are the ultimate Punk eye make-up. For the best result, choose a light colour, a deeper colour and an accent colour. Strong,*

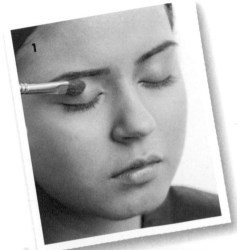

1 Using a medium-sized fluffy eye-shadow brush, apply a wash of light mauve eye-shadow over the entire lid, before blending it outwards and upwards towards to the brow bone.

**2** Using a darker purple eye-shadow and a firmer flat brush with an angled end to give you precision, create an inverted V-shape at the outer corner of the eye. Do this by drawing a diagonal line from the outer corner of the eye to the bottom of the eyebrow, and then take the colour under the brow bone towards the inner corner of the eye. Blend the colour inwards to soften the edges.

**3** Using the angled brush, outline the coloured area with a rich blue eye-shadow. This time, take the colour all the way along the lower lash line – you may find it easier to use a square-edged brush to do this. Blend the colour inwards, as before.

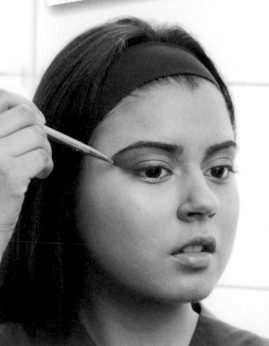

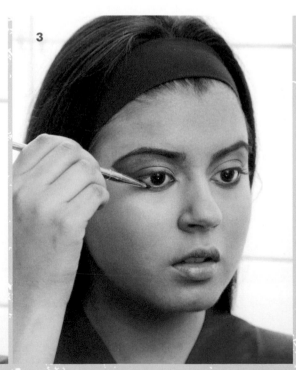

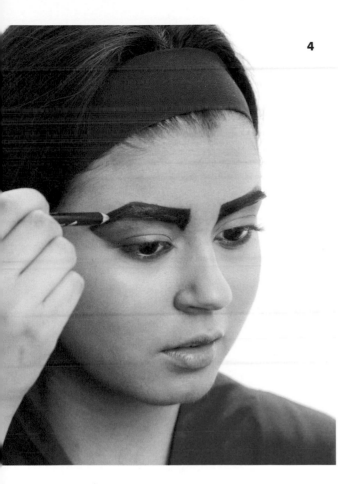

**4** Create sharp, exaggerated angular eyebrows using black or dark brown kohl pencil. Fill in your natural brows first and then take your time creating the shape to ensure that your finished eyebrows are perfectly symmetrical.

**5** For extra definition, you can use either a soft kohl pencil or a liquid eyeliner in bold blue to emphasize the top lash line and the inner rim of the lower lash line. Then finish with at least two coats of black mascara.

**5**

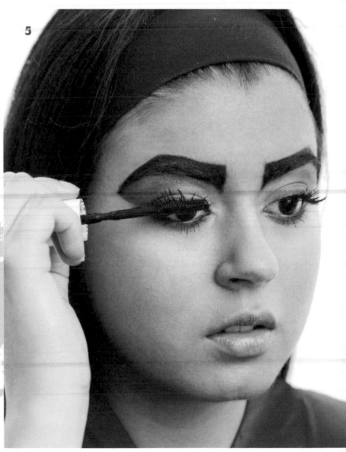

*For an authentic eighties look, apply a bold lipstick and emphasize your cheekbones with strong blusher.*

# Modern Mohawk

*If your hair isn't long enough to tie knots in the ponytails, just wrap a small section of hair around the base of each and secure it with hair grips/bobby pins.*

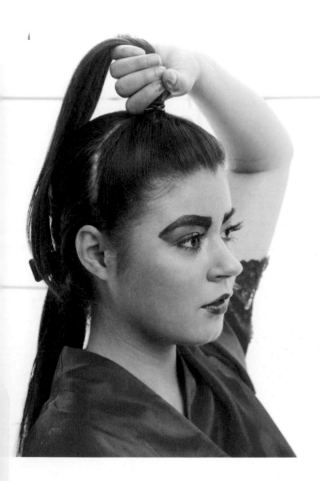 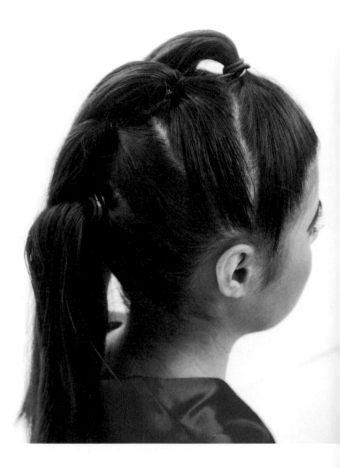

**1** This style is easiest to do if your hair has not just been washed. Work on dry hair and brush it through thoroughly before you start, using a natural-bristle hairbrush. Then, with a comb, draw a line from just in front of the top of your ear, across the top of your head and down to just in front of the top of your other ear. Comb this section of hair upwards and place it in a ponytail on top of your head. The section of hair should be about 5 cm/2 inches thick.

**2** In the same way, create a second section of hair of the same thickness behind the first. You should start drawing the parting just behind the top of your ear. Comb the hair upwards and place it in a ponytail in the centre of your head directly behind the first. Repeat this process to create four or five ponytails along the middle of the top of your head. Try to keep the sections neat and the same thickness to create symmetry in the finished look.

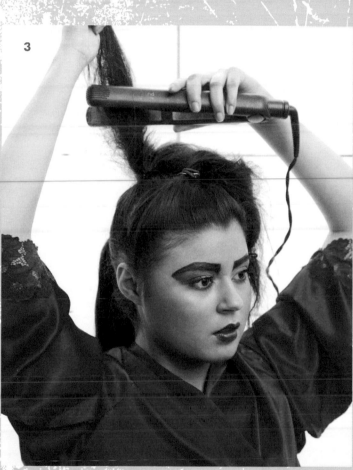

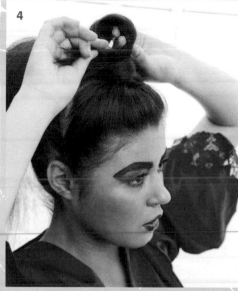

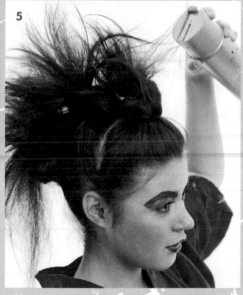

**3** Starting at the front and working back, backcomb the ends of the ponytails with a medium-tooth comb and apply a generous amount of hairspray through to the ends. Straighten these sections of hair with straightening irons, working from the roots to the ends along each length.

**4** Tie each section of hair into a knot at the base of each individual ponytail, pulling the ends through. Secure the knots to the head with hair grips/bobby pins all the way along.

**5** Fan out the ends of each ponytail to create a Mohawk effect, teasing the hair into shape with the comb and your fingers. Finish with plenty of hairspray to ensure the style keeps its shape. If you wish, apply a wash-out colour spray of your choice.

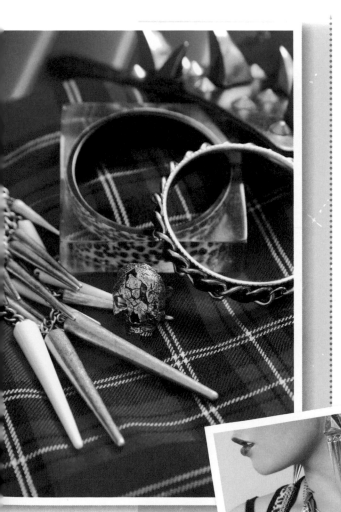

### gloves

Lace, leather and PVC were hugely popular materials during the 1980s and so occasion or dress gloves made a comeback. Fingerless gloves, or 'glovelettes', proved popular, as you could maintain more dexterity than with full-finger gloves while still rocking the latest fashion.

### piercings & tattoos

Not for the faint-hearted, piercings and tattoos are visual statements that require commitment. Nowadays, however, good-quality fake piercings and a wealth of temporary tattoo designs give you a chance to wear a look and see if you can live with it. There are also tattoo sleeves – essentially, patterned flexible mesh tubes – which you can wear on your arms and remove at the end of the day.

### studs, pins & ripped clothes

The Punk movement had a strong disaffection for conformity and this was no better reflected than by the wearing of ripped garments held together with safety pins. Before you go about ripping items, assess the type of material, as some items will instantly fray and become impossible to work with. Consider customizing denim with studs, safety pins and kilt pins, as well as stitching on slogan patches and scraps of tartan fabric. Skin-tight jeans were often splashed with bleach or adorned with chains.

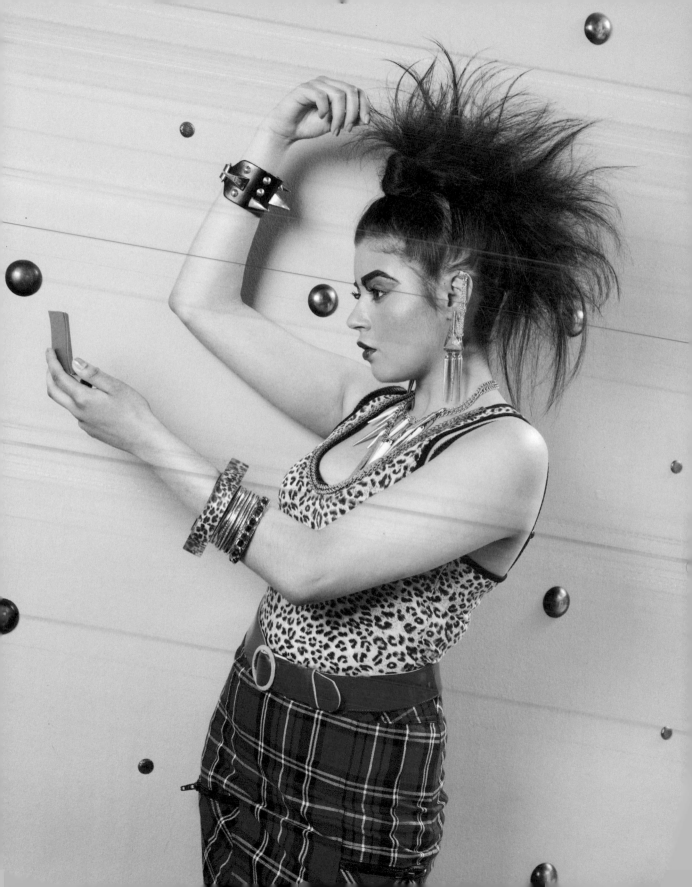

# HAIR TOOLS

*The selection of hair tools and products available in the modern marketplace is vast and, often, what works best for one individual may differ from the next. For that reason, it is always a good idea to experiment, if possible, before making an investment. Below is a selection of tools that tend to work for most and which I recommend you have in your vintage hairstyling kit.*

### HAIR PINS/GRIPS

Often referred to as Kirby grips or bobby pins, metal hair pins were popularized in the early 1920s when they were used to hold the newly fashionable bobbed hairstyles in place. They come in a variety of sizes and colours and should be matched as closely as possible to your hair colour in order to hold styles invisibly. Decorative hair pins are pretty way to finish a look.

### ROLLERS

Available in a range of sizes, rollers are cylindrical barrels around which sections of hair are wrapped to create curls (see page 14). They can be used on a variety of hair lengths and textures. An early, cost-effective method of curling hair was 'rag-rolling', which entailed wrapping sections of damp hair around strips of material and leaving it to dry. In recent years, bendy rollers, heated rollers and velcro rollers have been created and are an essential part of a vintage hairstyling kit.

### HAIRDRYER

The earliest hairdryers were developed from vacuum cleaners and the first electric hairdryer was patented in 1890 by Alexandre Godefoy. Over the years, we have come to be educated on the damage that the prolonged application of heat can have on our hair, so a good hairdryer should have a combination of heat settings and a high power rating to reduce the length of time needed to dry your hair or set a style.

### DRYING HOOD

Although not designed to make you look attractive when using it, the drying hood is the perfect tool for home hairstyling using rollers. After setting your hair in rollers, a drying hood can be placed over your hair and fastened under your chin.

A hairdryer is inserted into a tube attached to the hood, which concentrates and contains the heat over your curls. With the cool air setting on your hairdryer, you are able to set your hair in a much quicker time frame.

## A SELECTION OF COMBS

Combs are among the oldest tools found by archaeologists, having been discovered in very refined forms from settlements dating back more than 5,000 years. They have two main uses – to detangle hair and to assist in styling. I recommend that the minimum number of combs you have in your home hairstyling kit is three: a pin-tail comb for sectioning and backcombing, a medium-tooth comb for smoothing and styling, and a wide-tooth comb for combing wet hair without breaking it.

## STRAIGHTENING IRONS AND CURLING IRONS

Humans have always coveted that which they do not have, and within the world of beauty the desire for curly hair or straight hair by those born with the opposite is by no means a modern predisposition. Early curling irons were developed as long ago as 1866, with straightening irons, or 'flat irons', following in 1909. Modern commercial irons are available with varying barrel sizes to create different results and to suit different hair lengths, so it is important to take into consideration your hair length prior to purchase. (See page 15.)

## HAIR PADDING

An essential piece of kit for structuring hairstyles including beehives and buns, hair padding – most typically synthetic material fashioned into a sausage or donut shape – can be purchased with relative ease. However, it is not difficult to create your own cost-efficient padding using an old pair of stockings or tights/pantyhose. Cut one of the legs near the foot, approximately where the ankle would be, and stuff the stocking with net until it is the desired size. Tie a knot in the end and use accordingly. (See page 16.)

# MAKE-UP TOOLS

*There is no definitive right or wrong when it comes to make-up application methods, but certain tools will, about the type of your products as well as giving you greater accuracy in product placement.*

## BRUSHES

Available in synthetic and natural hair, the quality of your brushes will make a significant difference to how well your make-up blends and its ultimate finish on your skin. Natural-hair brushes are made from a variety of sources:

## PONY

Typically used for blusher brushes and various eye-shadow blending brushes, pony hair falls at the less expensive end of the scale.

## BADGER

Coarse in texture and great for applying defining eye-shadow and for filling brows, badger hair is widely used in an array of brush types and is relatively inexpensive.

## SQUIRREL

Expensive and less widely available, squirrel hair is fabulous used in brushes designed for blending.

## GOAT (CAPRA)

The most expensive natural-hair brushes, but, in my opinion, worth splashing out on, goat-hair is extremely soft and is perfect for the smooth application of foundation.

## MINK (KOLINSKY)

The flexibility of the hairs combined with an ultra-fine tip allow for precision in the placement of gel or liquid eyeliner. Given that eyeliner application is one of the most difficult techniques to master, I believe the high price often charged for this type of brush is justified.

## SABLE

Like badger hair, sable is widely used in the manufacture of cosmetics brushes. Less coarse than badger, it is softer on the face and falls within the medium cost range.

## SYNTHETIC BRUSHES

Largely made up from polyester or nylon fibres, synthetic brushes provide an alternative for individuals with sensitivities and allergies to animal hair. They are typically much rougher on the skin than natural-hair alternatives, but are often preferred due to their inexpensive price tag. There are other benefits, too. Synthetic fibres don't absorb pigments and chemicals, which natural hairs do, making them prone to damage unless they are looked after properly. They also provide a substitute for those who object to natural-hair brushes on moral grounds, although it is now possible to choose ethically sourced materials.

## CARING FOR YOUR BRUSHES

Whatever your brushes are made from, treat them as you would your own hair. Wash them regularly with a good shampoo to prevent a build-up of product and dirt, condition them and rinse thoroughly. Never stand wet brushes up in a pot or make-up belt to dry; water will seep downwards into the handles and become a breeding ground for bacteria. Dry your brushes with a hairdryer, directing the flow of air in the same direction as the hairs to prevent them from splaying.

## PRODUCTS AND RECOMMENDED MAKE-UP KIT

The variety of products available can be overwhelming, so below is my recommended make-up kit. Due to the ingredients, many products have a shelf life within which time they should be used – this ranges from between three months (mascara) and 36 months (eye-shadow and lipstick). My advice is to label new cosmetics with the date of purchase, so you can keep track and discard them accordingly.

Brushes – foundation, eye-shadow definer, eye-shadow fluff/blending, eyeliner, round-edge blusher, lip, brow.
Tools – tweezers, pencil sharpener, false lashes, lash glue.
Products – eye-shadow palette (six to eight colours suitable for your skin tone), kohl pencil and gel eyeliner/liquid eyeliner, black or brown mascara, two to three foundation colours (blend the perfect colour to match your skin tone as it alters through the seasons), primer, concealer, highlighter, bronzer, brow powder, blusher, lipstick, lip liner, lip gloss, setting powder.

# UK SOURCES

**Spitalfields Market**
www.visitspitalfields.com
78 Quaker Street
London E1 6SW

An eclectic selection of shops and markets selling new and vintage clothing.

**Camden Passage Market**
www.camdenpassageislington.co.uk
Islington
London N1 5ED

Shops, arcades and markets selling vintage clothing and homewares.

**Vivien Of Holloway**
www.vivienofholloway.com
294 Holloway Road
London N7 6NJ

The very best of 1940s and 1950s reproduction clothing and accessories.

**Alfies Antique Market**
www.alfiesantiques.com
13-25 Church Street
London NW8 8DT

A large indoor market selling a wide range of antiques, from clothing to furniture.

**What Katie Did**
www.whatkatiedid.com
26 Portobello Green
London W10 5TZ

Specialists in vintage lingerie, hosiery, swimwear and accessories.

**Rokit**
www.rokit.co.uk
225 Camden High Street
London NW1 7BU

Second hand vintage clothing and accessories from the 1940s to the 1980s.

**Beyond Retro**
www.beyondretro.com
110-112 Cheshire Street
London E2 6EJ

A second hand vintage clothing retailer based in London and Brighton.

**London Vintage Store**
www.londonvintagestore.com
162 Holloway Road
London N7 8DQ

Second hand vintage clothing and accessories from the 1940s to the 1990s.

**Ribbons & Taylor**
www.ribbonsandtaylor.co.uk
157 Stoke Newington
Church Street
London N16 0UH

Glamorous vintage clothing and costume for men and women.

**Berty & Gerty**
www.bertyandgerty.co.uk
41 Inverness Street
Camden Town
London NW1 8AF

An eclectic mix of vintage clothing and accessories.

**What Goes Around Comes Around**
Mezzanine 3
The Stables Market
Chalk Farm Road
London NW1 8AH

Purveyors of vintage clothing, accessories and bicycles.

**Absolute Vintage**
www.absolutevintage.co.uk
15 Hanbury Street
London E1 6QR

High-quality vintage clothing and accessories.

**The Vintage Showroom**
www.thevintageshowroom.com
14 Earlham Street
London WC2H 9LN

Specialists in vintage menswear and tailoring.

**Afflecks**
www.afflecks.com
52 Church Street
Manchester M4 1PW

A vast emporium of vintage eclecticism.

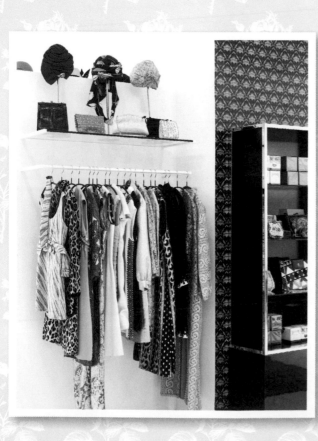

# US SOURCES

**Pop Boutique**
www.pop-boutique.com
58 Whitechapel
Liverpool
Merseyside L1 6EG

*Recycled vintage and retro
clothes from the 1950s to
the 1980s.*

**Now, Voyager**
www.now-voyager.co.uk
17 Market Place
Southend-on-Sea
Essex SS1 1DA

*Specialists in vintage-
style fascinators and
hair accessories.*

**Snoopers Paradise**
7 Kensington Gardens
North Laine
Brighton BN1 4AL

*A wide range of antique
furniture, clocks, paintings
and homewares.*

**Vintage at Number 18**
www.vintageatnumber18
.co.uk
18A Blandford Square
Newcastle
Tyne and Wear NE1 4HZ

*A vintage boutique selling
clothing and accessories
for women.*

**Mama's Vintage &
Antiques Boutique**
The Tower
Uptin House
Newcastle
Tyne and Wear NE2 1TZ

*Original and vintage-
inspired clothing, books,
music and homewares.*

**Cox and Baloney**
www.coxandbaloney.com
182 Cheltenham Road
Bristol BS6 5RB

*Original and vintage-
inspired clothing,
accessories and furniture.*

**Uncle Sam's American
Vintage Clothing**
www.unclesamsamericanvin
tage.weebly.com
54A Park Street
Bristol
Somerset BS1 5JN

*Vintage clothing imported
directly from the USA.*

**Vintage at Madisons**
1 Canal Road
Tavistock
Devon PL19 8AR

*Vintage clothing, antique
and costume jewellery and
vintage accessories*

**Cheap Jack's**
www.cheapjacks.com
303 5th Avenue
New York 10016

*The largest vintage clothing
store on the east coast.*

**Vintage Thrift Shop**
www.vintagethriftshop.org
286 3rd Avenue
New York 10010

*Vintage clothing,
accessories, furniture,
costume jewellery
and homewares.*

**New York Vintage**
www.newyorkvintage.com
117 West 25th Street
New York 10001

*Specialists in vintage
couture clothing
and antiques.*

**Star Struck Vintage
Clothing**
www.starstruckvintage.com
47 Greenwich Avenue
New York 10014

*Vintage treasures for men,
women and children.*

**Poor Little Rich Girl**
www.shoppoorlittlerichgirl
.com
121 Hampshire Street
Cambridge MA 02141

*Second hand and vintage
clothing and accessories.*

**Artifaktori**
www.artifaktori.com
22a College Avenue
Somerville MA 02144

*Vintage clothing, accessories
and other treasures.*

**Cambridge Antique
Market**
www.marketantique.com
201 Monsignor O'Brien
Highway
Cambridge MA 02141

*A large market selling
vintage clothing, books,
furniture and collectibles.*

**Palm Beach Vintage**
www.palmbeachvintage.com
3623 South Dixie Highway
West Palm Beach FL 33405

*Purveyors of couture and
fine vintage clothing.*

**Deja Vu Vintage Clothing**
1825 North Orange Avenue
Orlando FL 32804

*Premium vintage,
handmade and all things
one-of-a-kind.*

**Revolve Clothing
Exchange**
www.revolve.cx
1620 East 7th Avenue
Tampa FL 33605

*New and experienced
clothing, accessories,
jewellery, gifts and shoes.*

**Buffalo Exchange**
www.buffaloexchange.com
1521 Central Avenue
Charlotte NC 28205

*New and re-cycled clothing*
*for men and women.*

**Zenith Antiques**
www.zenithpgh.com
86 South 26th Street
Pittsburgh PA 15205

*An eclectic selection of*
*vintage clothing, antiques*
*and collectibles.*

**Iguana Vintage Clothing**
www.iguanaclothing.com
6320 Hollywood Boulevard
Los Angeles CA 90028

*Stylish vintage clothing*
*and accessories.*

**American Superior**
**Vintage**
www.americansuperior
vintageclothing.com
7277 Melrose Avenue
Los Angeles CA 90046

*Original vintage clothing*
*from the 1950s to the 1970s.*

**Sielian's Vintage Apparel**
www.sieliansvintageapparel.
com
9013 Melrose Avenue
West Hollywood CA 90069

*Sexy, form-fitting clothing*
*from the 1960s to the 1980s.*

**Everything's Jake**
www.jakevintage.com
4644 Hollywood Boulevard
Los Angeles CA 90027

*Vintage brands for the*
*modern gentleman.*

**Dolly Python**
www.dollypythonvintage.com
1916 North Haskell Avenue
Dallas TX 75204

*Multi award-winning*
*vintage emporium*

**Second Looks**
www.secondlooksaustin.com
8108 Mesa Drive
Austin TX 78759

*Upscale vintage clothing*
*for men.*

**Feathers Boutique**
www.feathersboutiquevinta
ge.blogspot.co.uk
1700 South Congress
Avenue
Austin TX 78704

*Vintage, new and vintage-*
*inspired adornments.*

**Stefan's Vintage Clothing**
www.stefansvintageclothing
.com
1160 Euclid Avenue
Northeast
Atlanta GA 30307

*Atlanta's oldest vintage*
*clothing store – fashion*
*from the 1900s to the 1970s.*

**Junction**
www.junctionwdc.com
1510 U Street Northwest
Washington DC 20009

*Vintage and contemporary*
*clothing and jewellery, gifts*
*home wares and accessories*
*from the 1930s to today.*

**Black Eyed Susie**
3443 14th Street Northwest
Washington DC 20010

*Second hand vintage*
*clothing for men*
*and women.*

**PollySue's Vintage Shop**
www.pollysues.com
6915 Laurel Avenue
Takoma Park MD 20912

*Fine vintage clothing from*
*the 1850s to the 1970s.*

**Nana**
www.nanadc.com
3068 Mount Pleasant Street
Northwest
Washington DC 20009

*Vintage-inspired*
*sustainably-made clothing.*

**Miss Pixie's**
www.misspixies.com
1626 14th Street
Northwest
Washington DC 20009

*Vintage furniture,*
*collectibles and ephemera.*

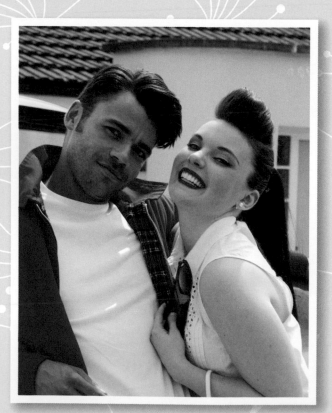

# PICTURE CREDITS

All photography by Penny Wincer apart from:

Caroline Arber page 72 insert.
Sandra Lane pages 28 above insert, 48 below insert,
80 above and below inserts.
Diana Miller backgrounds on pages 6, 7, 10, 12, 15,
16, 39, 45, 47, 48, 138, 139.
Claire Richardson page 48 above insert, page 61
above insert.
Polly Wreford page 112, 138 insert.

Illustrations
Page 21 © Victoria and Albert Museum, London.
Page 41 Mary Evans Picture Library/Peter & Dawn
Cope Collection.
Page 53 image courtesy of The Advertising
Archives.
Page 65 © Estate of David Wright/Mary Evans
Picture Library.
Page 85 image courtesy of Land of Lost Content
www.lolc.co.uk.
Page 97 image courtesy of The Advertising
Archives.
Page 117 image courtesy of Land of Lost Content
www.lolc.co.uk.

With special thanks to.
The Shoreditch (featured on pages 38 – 49) for
letting us use their beautiful location.
www.theshoreditch-london.com

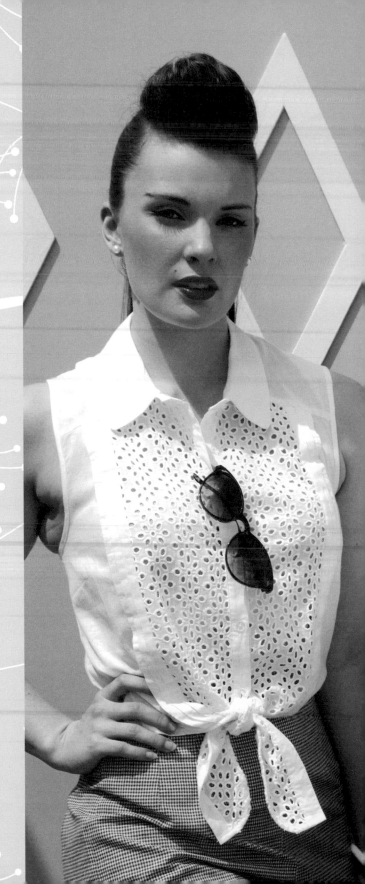

# INDEX

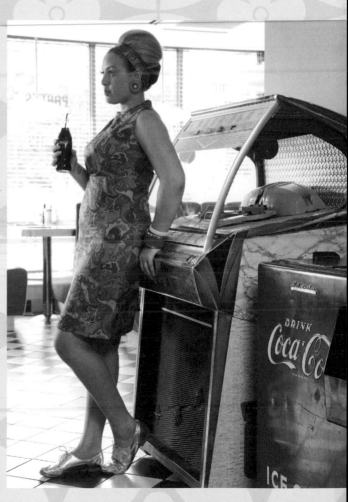

# ACKNOWLEDGEMENTS

With special thanks to the godfather of vintage, Wayne Hemingway, who selflessly took the time to mentor me – you are an inspiration. Special thanks also to Patricia and Ellen Bewley who kindly passed on their artistic genes, John Wing who tirelessly nurtured my passion for the past and my partner David Kuti, a staunch minimalist immersed in my baroque world.

Thanks to Katy Kendrick from Complete U for bringing the vintage hairstyling to life, Emma Goulding from Oh Sew Vintage www.ohsewvintage.co.uk for generously donating clothing from her beautiful reproduction vintage range, Dawn and Dave O'Gorman from The Little Shop for providing endless cups of tea and unlimited access to their amazing vintage stock, and Impet2us and Mary Quant Ltd for gifting a selection of products to use on my beautiful models.

Ryland Peters & Small would like to thank our wonderful models Alexandra, Amy, Beth, John, Lila, Nina, Sebastian, Tala and Veronica.

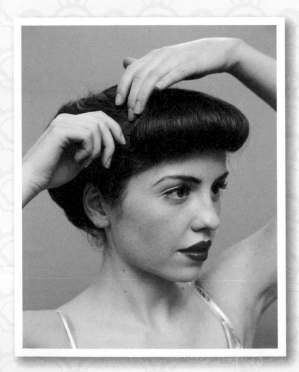

HSMIX +
E          HOLAB
Friends of the
Houston Public Library
HOLABIRD, KATHARINE
ANGELINA AT THE FAIR

02/05

HSMIX +
E
HOLAB

HOUSTON PUBLIC LIBRARY
SMITH

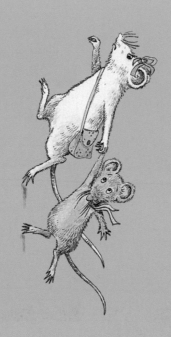

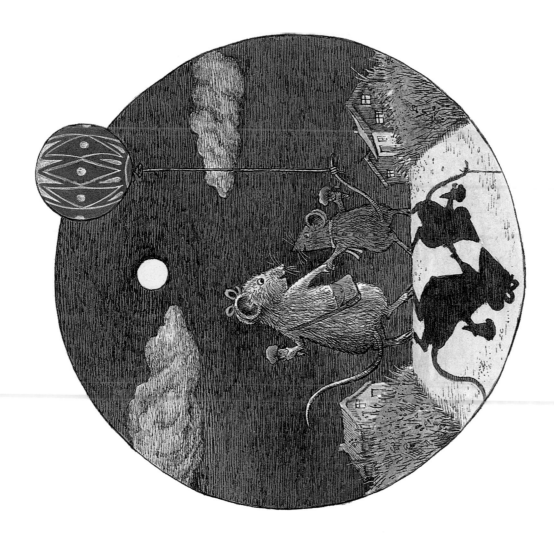

Afterward they had a double chocolate ice-cream cone and walked home slowly together. "I like fairs," said Henry, and Angelina smiled.

"You can come with me anytime," she said.

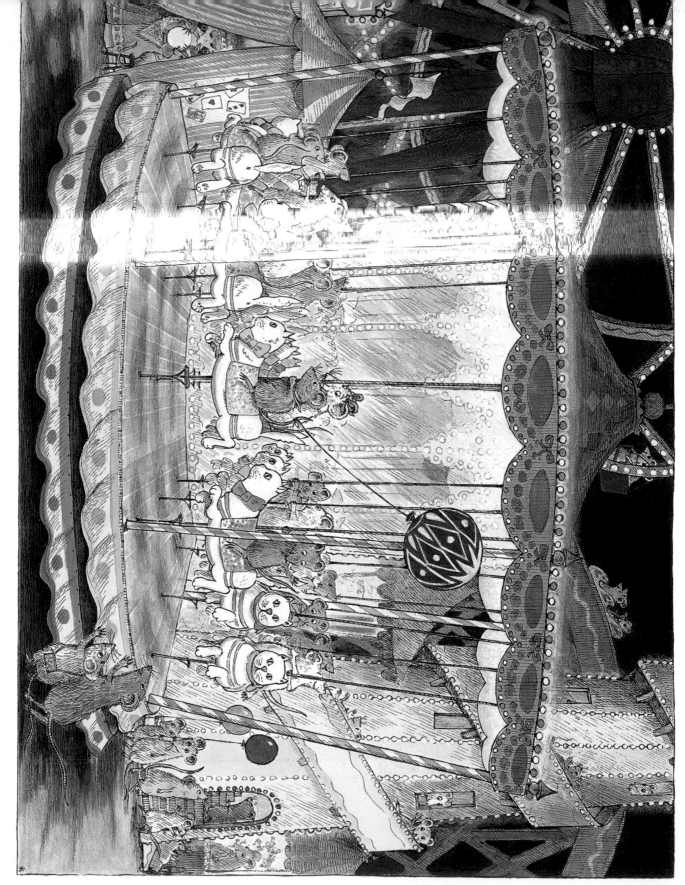

they went on three times, and they both loved it.

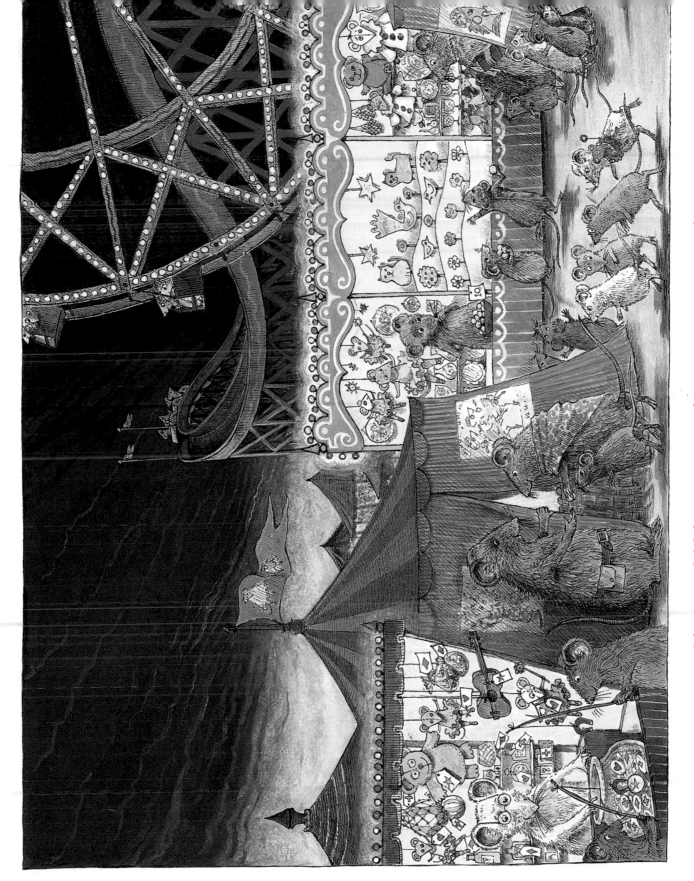

Henry said he would like to go on the merry-go-round,

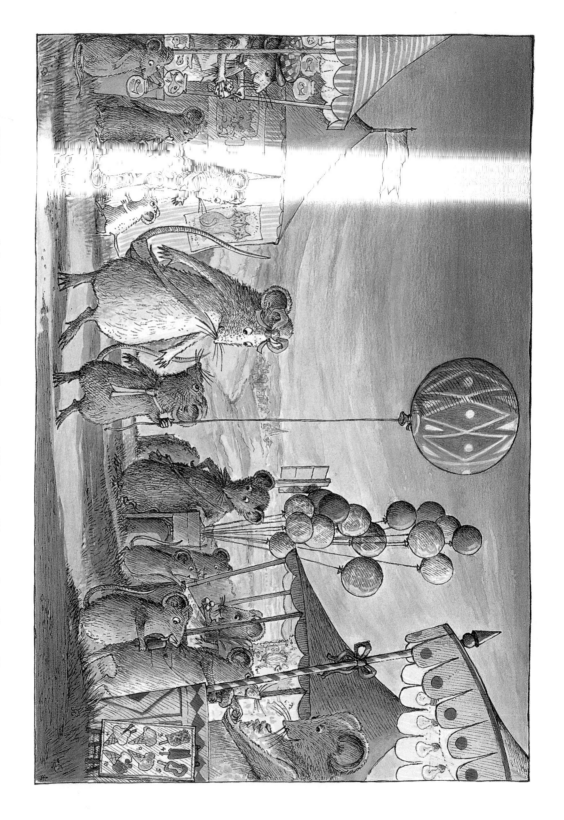

"What would you like to do now?" Angelina asked kindly.

And there, watching the balloon man blow up the beautiful balloons, was Henry! Angelina was so relieved that she gave him a big hug and a kiss.

"What is your favorite color, Henry?" she asked. Henry chose a blue balloon.

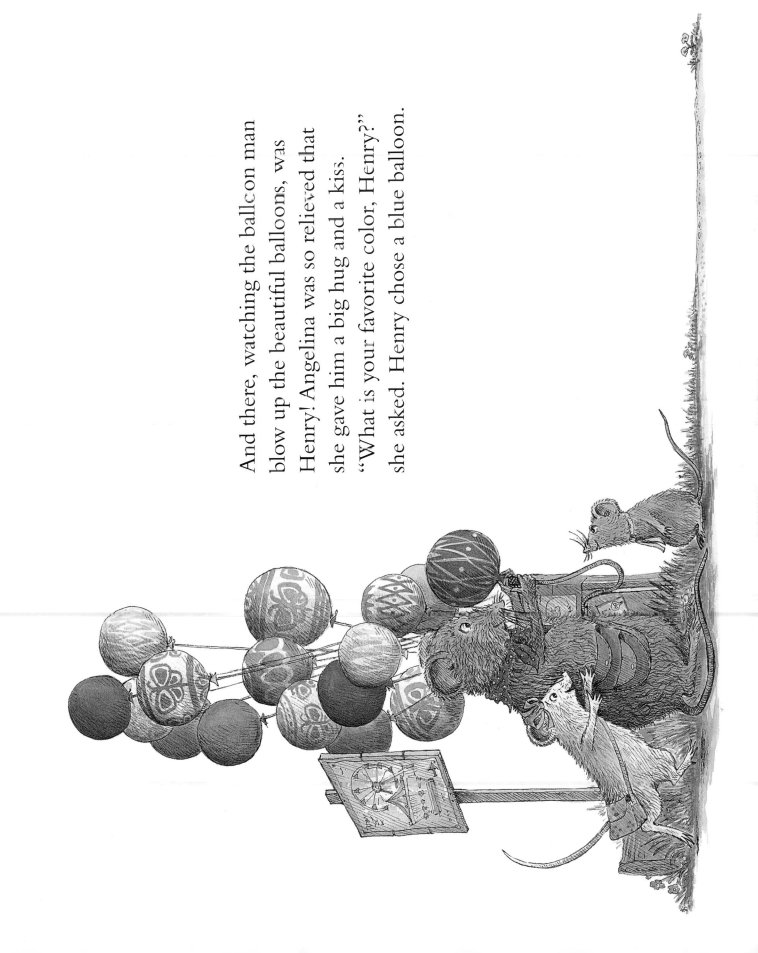

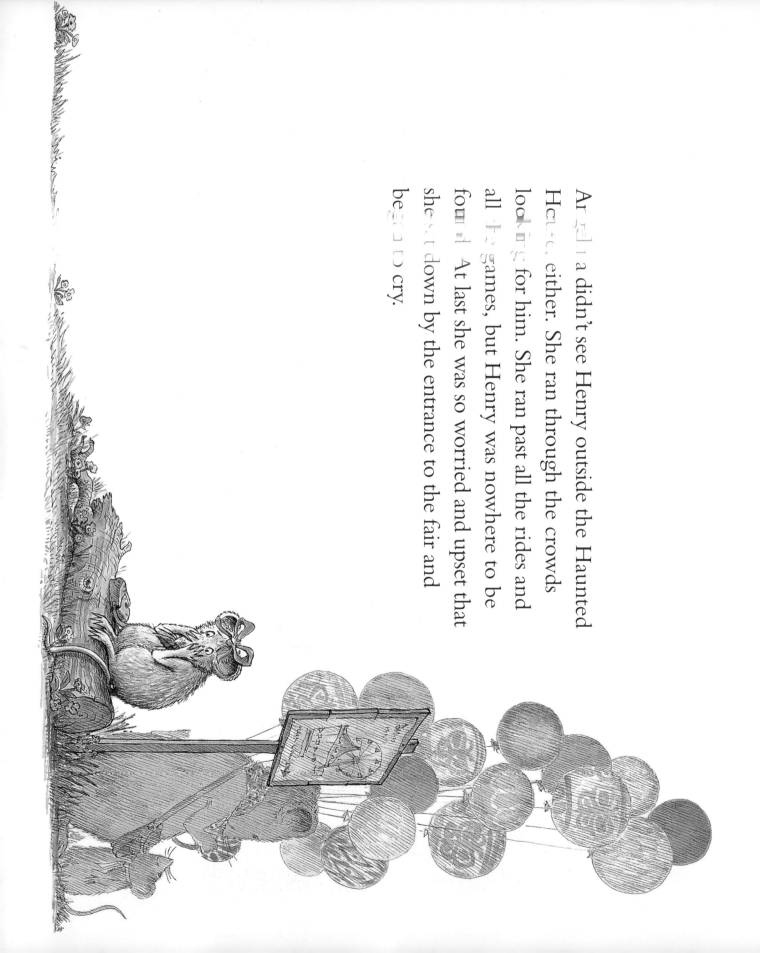

Angela didn't see Henry outside the Haunted House, either. She ran through the crowds looking for him. She ran past all the rides and all the games, but Henry was nowhere to be found. At last she was so worried and upset that she sat down by the entrance to the fair and began to cry.

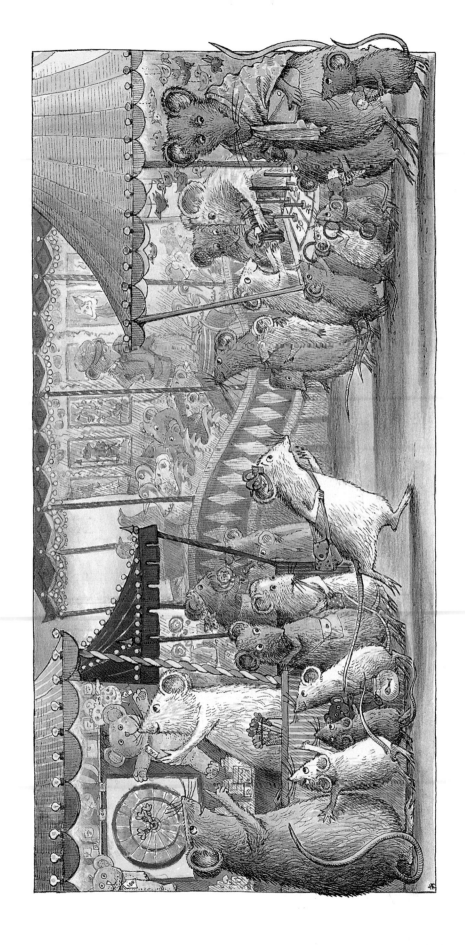

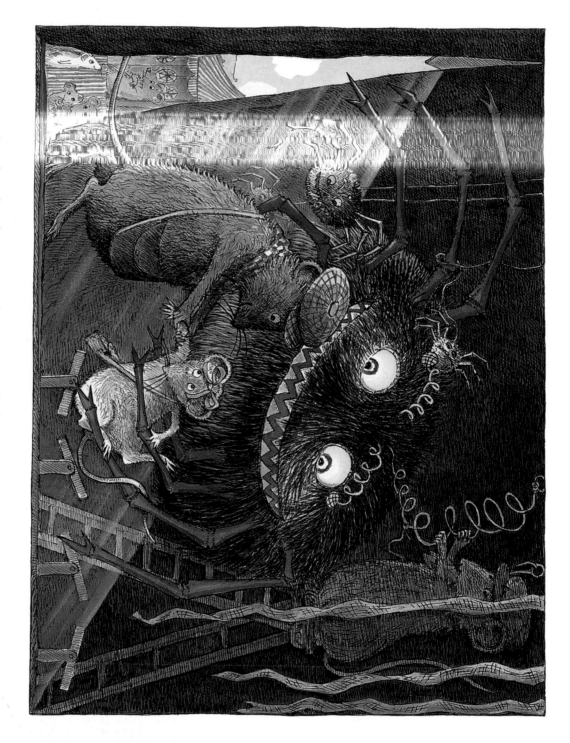

She looked everywhere until she got tangled up in the spider and had to be rescued by the ticket seller.

"Henry, Henry," Angelina called, but there was no answer in the darkness. Angelina hurried back through the Haunted House trying to find him.

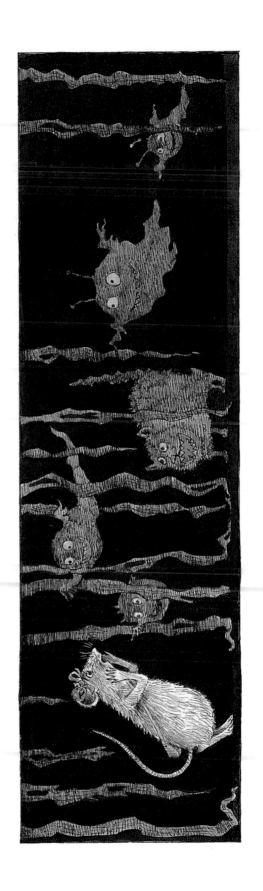

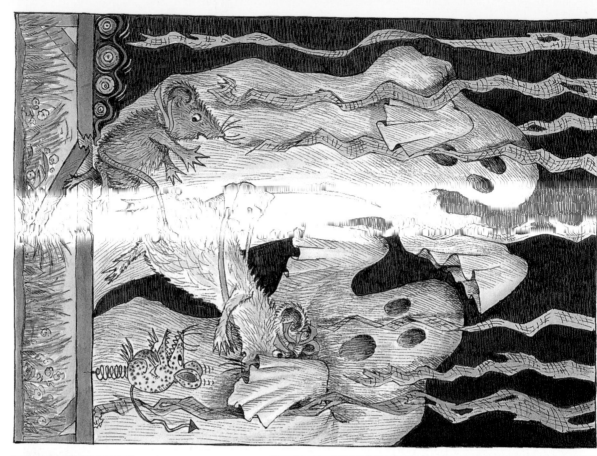

When they bumped into a ghost
Angelina reached out to touch Henry…

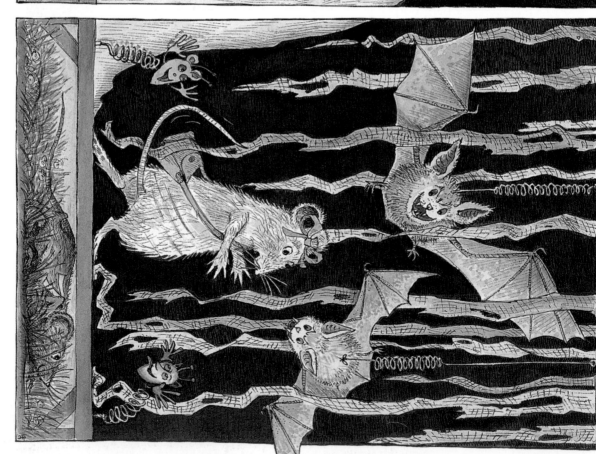

…but he was gone!

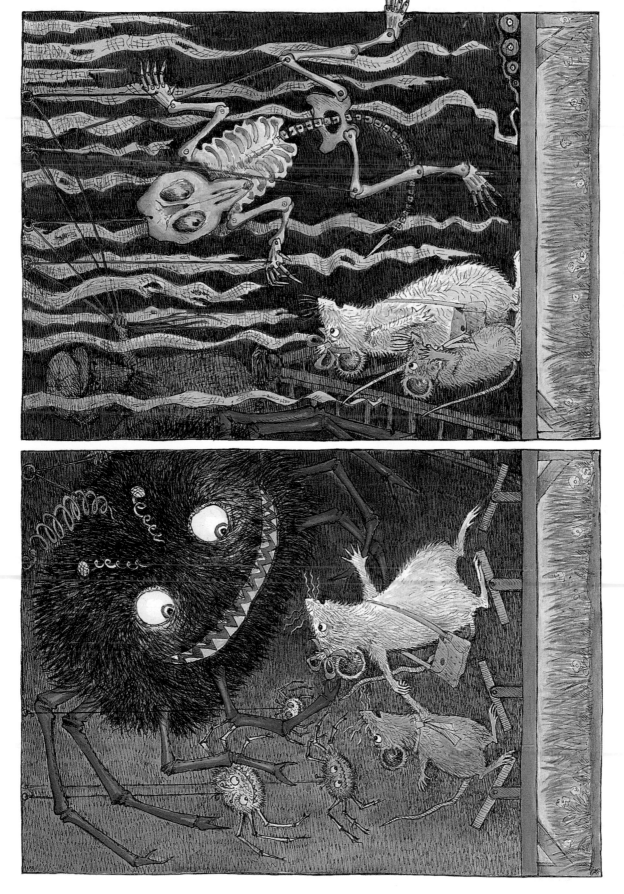

...and a skeleton jumped out and pointed right at them.

A big spider dangled just above their heads as they went in...

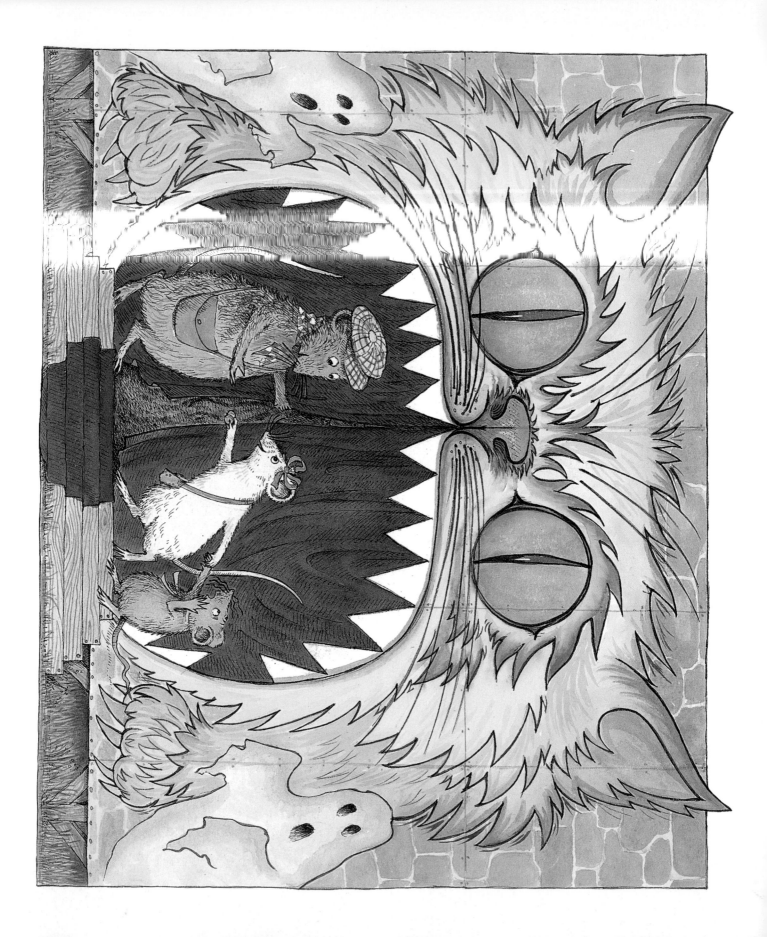

Then Angelina saw the Haunted House.

"You'll like this," she said, and pulled Henry inside.

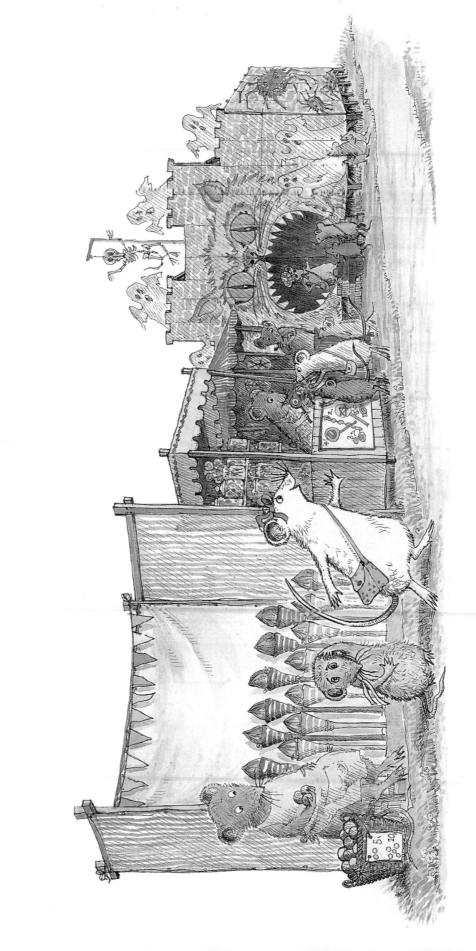

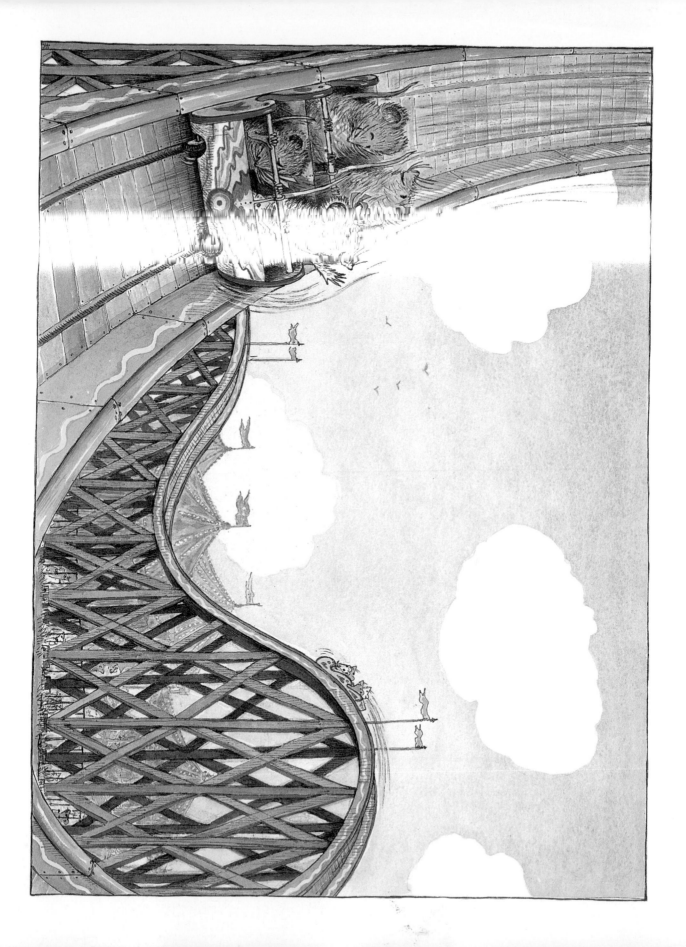

When they got off Henry felt sick, but he cheered up when he saw the merry-go-round. "Look!" he said. "Can we go on that?"

"Not now," said Angelina. "We're going on the fast rides." She took poor Henry on the roller coaster. Henry shut his eyes and held on tightly as the little car zoomed up and down the tracks. Angelina loved it and wanted to go again, but Henry wasn't sure he wanted to take any more rides at all.

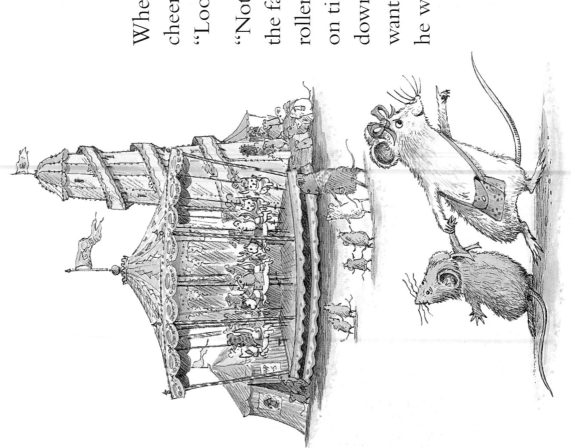

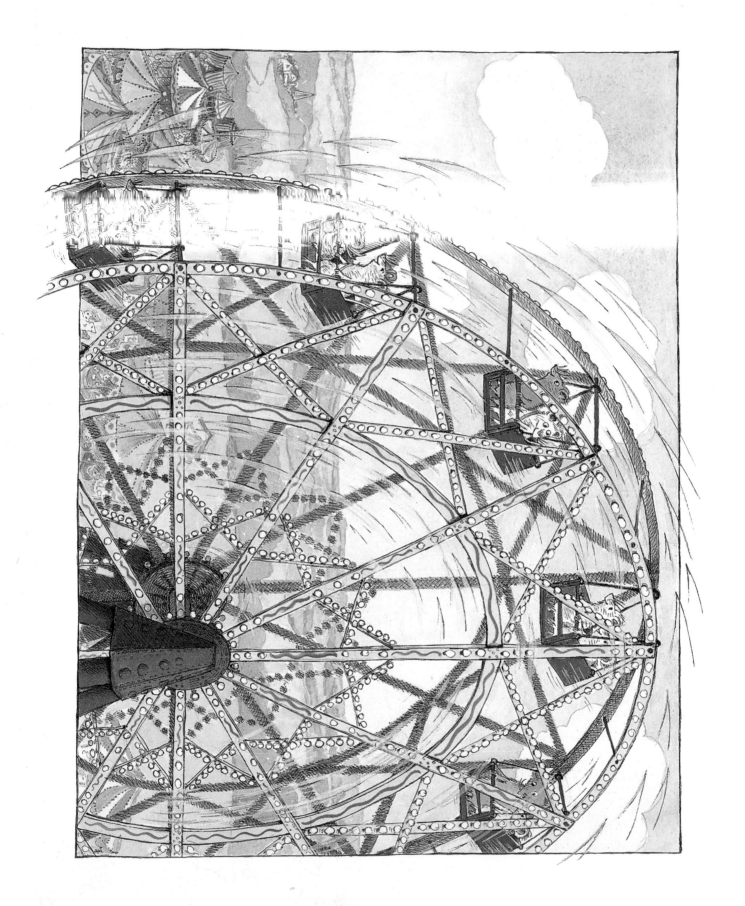

At the entrance to the fair was a stand of brightly colored balloons. "Oh, look!" cried Henry. "Balloons!"

But Angelina didn't pay any attention. "We're going on the Ferris wheel," she said. The Ferris wheel was huge and Henry was frightened, but Angelina loved the feeling of soaring up in the air, and so they took two rides.

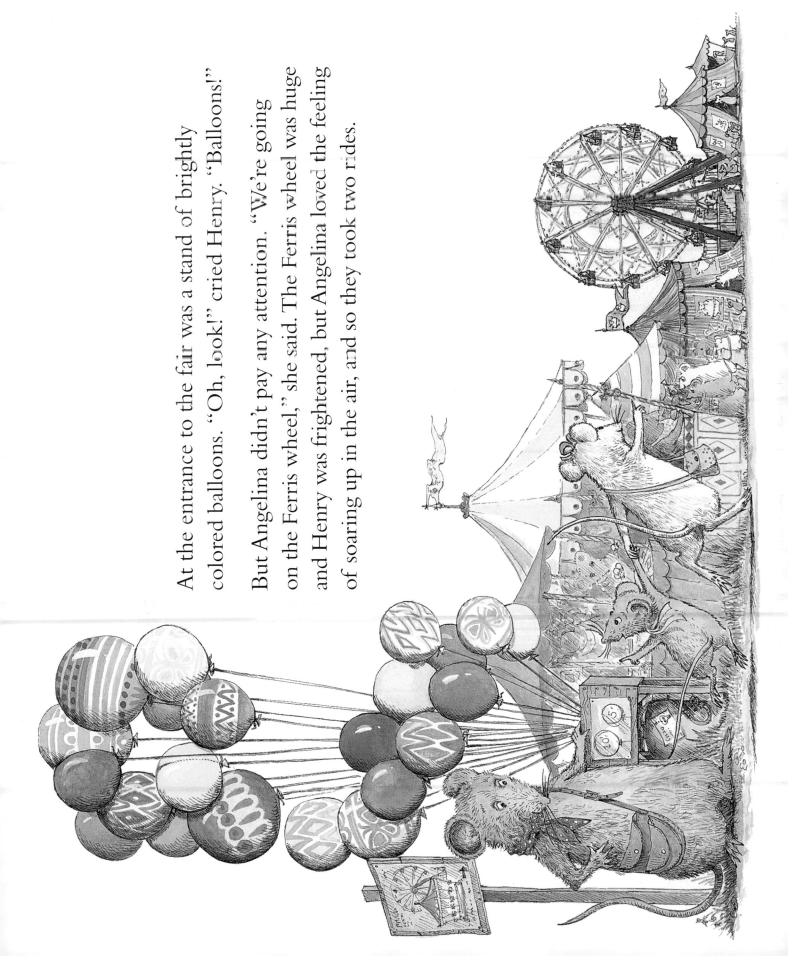

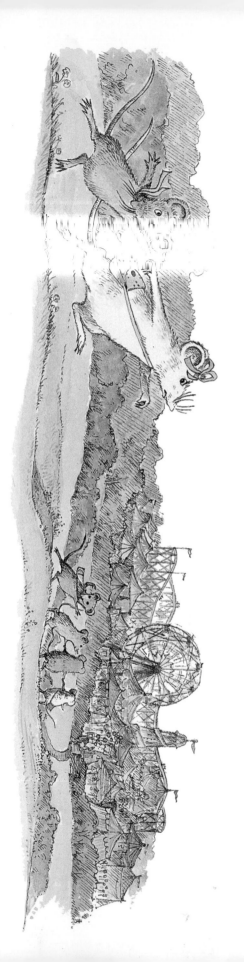

After the dance Angelina was ready to go to the fair with her friends, but her parents stopped her. "You've forgotten that little cousin Henry is visiting today," said Angelina's father. "He will be very disappointed if he can't go to the fair with you."

Angelina was furious. "I don't want to take Henry!" she said. "I hate little boys!" But Henry held out his hand just the same, and Angelina had to take him with her. The music from the fair was already floating across the fields, and Angelina's friends had gone ahead. She grabbed Henry's hand and dragged him along behind her, running as fast as she could.

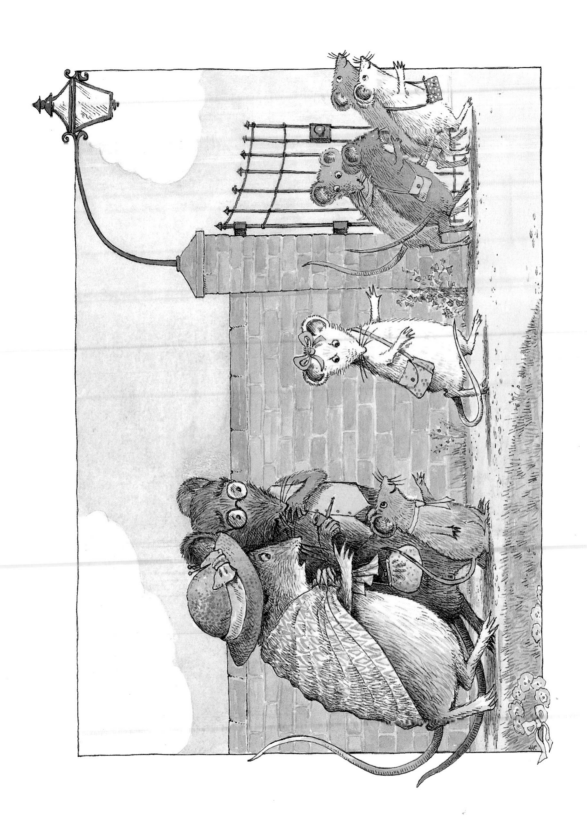

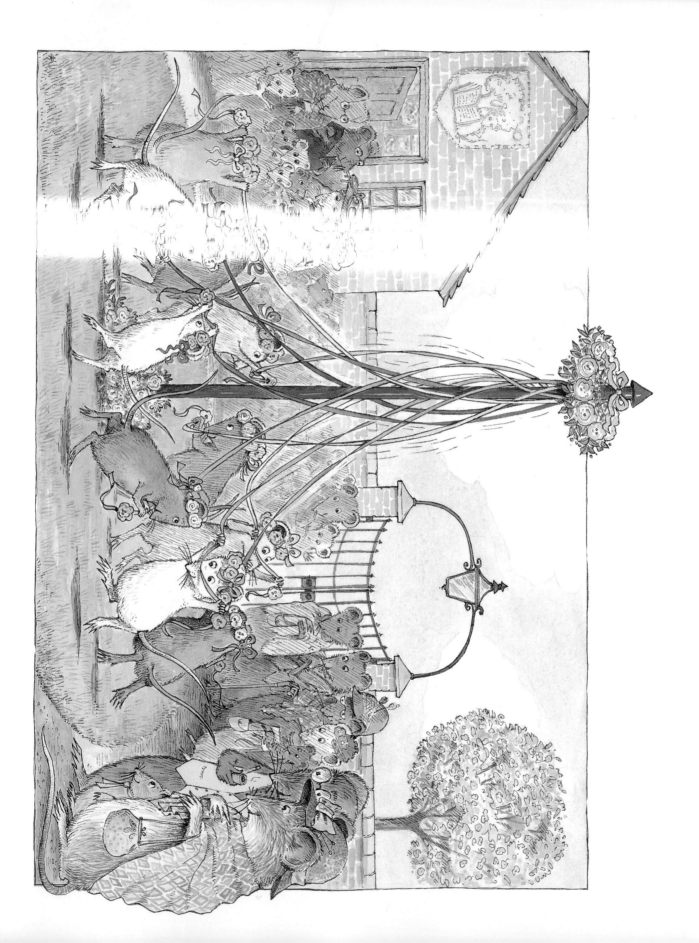

At last, when all the snow had melted, and the wind was soft and warm again, the May Day Fair arrived in town. Angelina's ballet class performed a maypole dance at school in celebration of spring, and Angelina almost flew around the maypole she was so excited. All the parents watched and cheered.

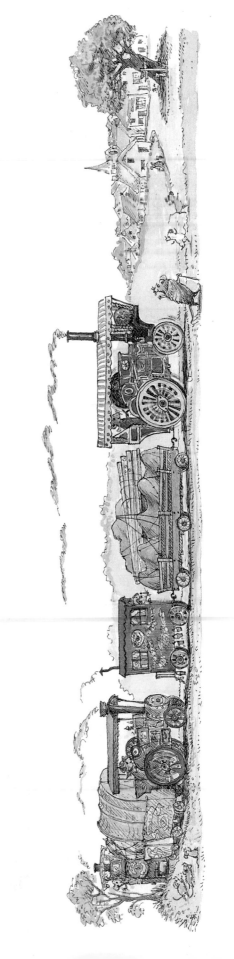

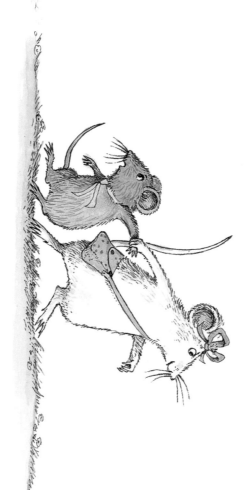

# Angelina
## at the Fair

Katharine Holabird

Illustrations by Helen Craig

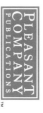

PLEASANT COMPANY PUBLICATIONS ™

*For Tara, Alexandra and Adam    KH*
*To Ben and Vitti with Love    HC*

Published by Pleasant Company Publications
© 2000 HIT Entertainment PLC
Text copyright © 1985 Katharine Holabird
Illustrations copyright © 1985 Helen Craig

All rights reserved. No part of this book may be used or reproduced in any manner whatsoever without written permission except in the case of brief quotations embodied in critical articles and reviews.
For information, address: Book Editor, Pleasant Company Publications, 8400 Fairway Place, P.O. Box 620998, Middleton, Wisconsin 53562.

Visit our Web site at www.americangirl.com

Second Edition
Printed in Italy.
00 01 02 03 04 05 06 LEGO 10 9 8 7 6 5 4 3 2

Library of Congress Cataloging-in-Publication Data
Craig, Helen.
Angelina at the fair / illustrations by Helen Craig ; story by Katharine Holabird.
    p. cm.
Summary: Angelina's annoyance at having to take her little cousin Henry to the fair turns into friendship after a day filled with adventures and surprises.
ISBN 1-58485- 44-9
[1. Fairs—Fiction. 2. Cousins—Fiction. 3. Mice—Fiction.]
I. Holabird, Katharine. II. Title.
PZ7.C84418 Amd 2000
[E]—dc21    00-022880

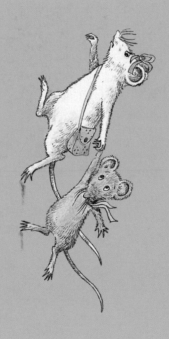

D060245

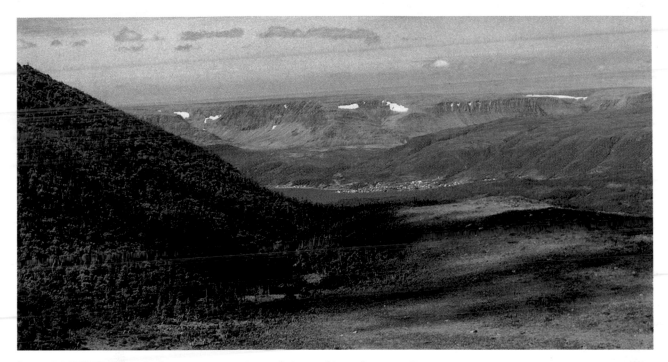

because the overwhelming majority of Canadians live within 100 miles (160 kilometers) of the U.S. border, in practical terms the nation is long and skinny. We are in fact an archipelago of population islands separated by implacable barriers—the angry ocean, three mountain walls, and the Canadian Shield, that vast desert of billion-year-old rock that sprawls over half the country, rich in mineral treasures, impossible for agriculture.

Canada's geography makes the country difficult to govern and explains our obsession with transportation and communication. The government has to be involved in railways, airlines, and broadcasting networks as it is with social services such as universal medical care. Rugged individualism is not a Canadian quality. Given the environment, people long ago learned to work together for security.

It is ironic that the very bulwarks that separate us—the chiseled peaks of the Selkirk Mountains, the gnarled scarps north of Lake Superior, the ice-choked waters of Northumberland Strait —should also be among our greatest attractions for tourists and artists. But if that is the paradox of Canada, it is also the glory.

Newfoundland's Gros Morne National Park—a wilderness of woodlands, moors, and rugged coastal cliffs—epitomizes the austere beauty of Canada's easternmost province.

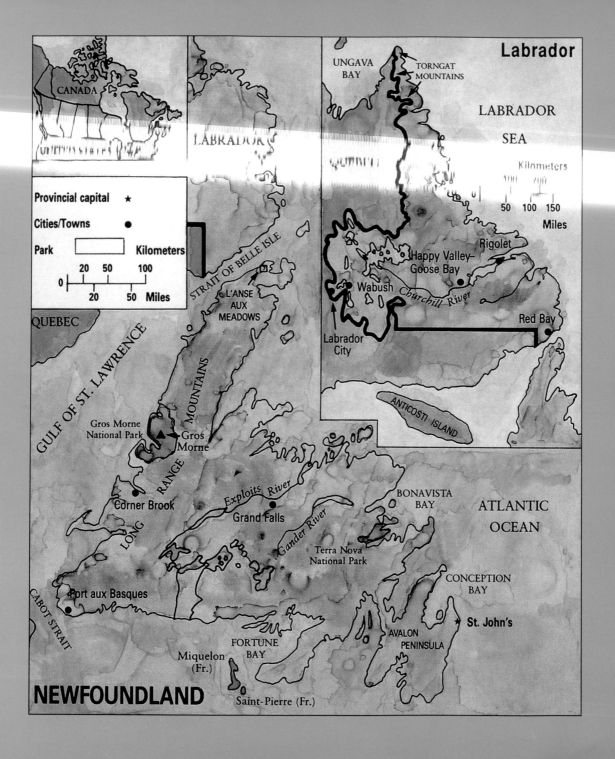

Labrador

UNGAVA BAY

TORNGAT MOUNTAINS

LABRADOR SEA

LABRADOR

CANADA

UNITED STATES

Rigolet

Happy Valley–Goose Bay

Wabush

Churchill River

Labrador City

Red Bay

Kilometers

50 100 150

Miles

Provincial capital ★

Cities/Towns ●

Park ☐

Kilometers

0    20   50   100

0         20        50    Miles

STRAIT OF BELLE ISLE

L'ANSE AUX MEADOWS

QUEBEC

GULF OF ST. LAWRENCE

Gros Morne National Park

Gros Morne

LONG RANGE MOUNTAINS

Corner Brook

Exploits River

Grand Falls

Gander River

Terra Nova National Park

BONAVISTA BAY

ATLANTIC OCEAN

CONCEPTION BAY

ANTICOSTI ISLAND

Port aux Basques

CABOT STRAIT

Miquelon (Fr.)

FORTUNE BAY

Saint-Pierre (Fr.)

AVALON PENINSULA

St. John's

NEWFOUNDLAND

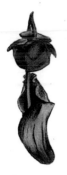
**Pitcher plant**

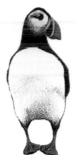
**Puffin**

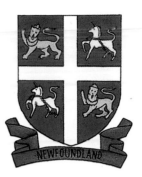

# Newfoundland at a Glance

**Area:** 156,185 square miles (404,519 square kilometers)

**Population:** 541,000 (1996 census)

**Capital:** St. John's (population 101,936)

**Other cities:** Corner Brook (population 21,893), Labrador City (population 8,455), Happy Valley—Goose Bay (population 8,655)

**Major rivers:** Churchill, Exploits

**Principal products:** Fish, forestry products, iron ore, hydroelectric power

**Entered Dominion of Canada:** March 31, 1949

**Motto:** *Quaerite prime regnum dei* (Seek ye first the Kingdom of God)

**Provincial coat of arms:** Red shield with white cross, two lions to represent England, and two unicorns to represent Scotland, with Native Canadians on either side and an elk on top of the shield; created in 1637, adopted in 1928

**Provincial flag:** Red, white, and blue design based upon the Union Jack, the flag of Great Britian; adopted in 1980

**Government:** Parliamentary system with a single-chambered legislature; 48 legislative representatives are popularly elected by district for terms of 5 years; the formal head of state is the lieutenant governor, appointed by Canada's federal government as representative of the British Crown; the head of government is the premier, leader of the dominant political party; the premier appoints an executive council from the legislative assembly; Newfoundland is represented in the federal government in Ottawa by 5 senators and 6 members of the House of Commons

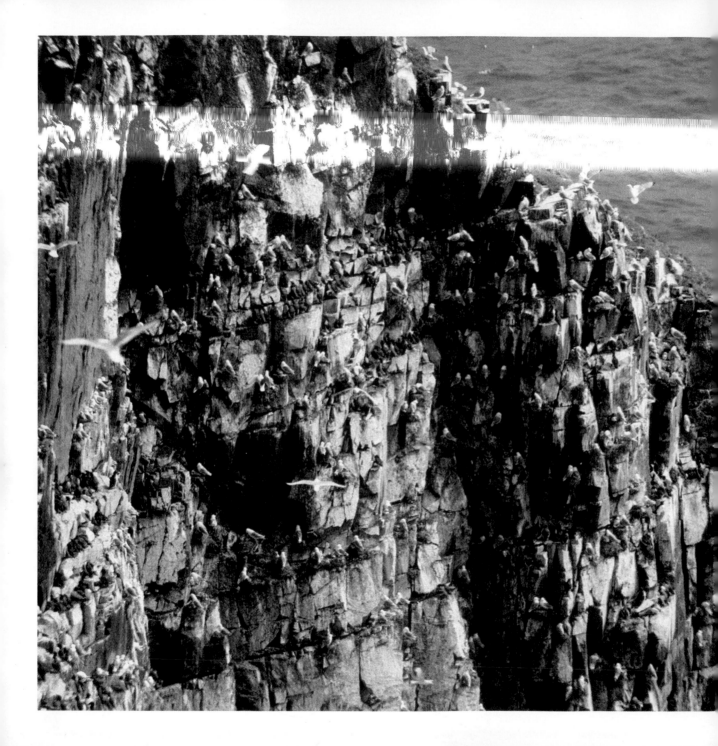

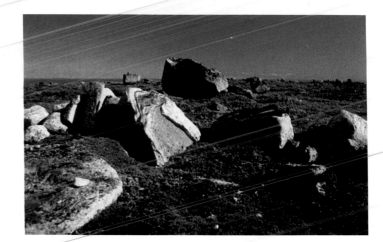

# The Land

Perhaps more than any other province in Canada, Newfoundland is defined by its relationship with the sea. The province consists of two parts, the island of Newfoundland and the region called Labrador on the Canadian mainland. The two are separated by a channel called the Strait of Belle Isle, and both the island and Labrador have long, rugged seacoasts. The fishing grounds that surround the island—among the most productive in the world— have shaped the province's history and economy.

Newfoundland is the largest of Canada's four Atlantic provinces; the others are Prince Edward Island, Nova Scotia, and New Brunswick. Although larger than the other three Atlantic provinces combined, Newfoundland accounts for little more than four percent of Canada's total land area. It is the seventh largest Canadian province in area and the ninth largest in population. Its overall area is 156,185 square miles (404,519 square kilometers). Mainland Labrador, with an area of 112,826 square miles (292,219 square kilometers), is more than two and one half times as large as the island of Newfoundland, which has an area of 43,359 square miles (112,300 square kilometers).

*Opposite:* Cape St. Mary's, on the Avalon Peninsula of Newfoundland island, is a bird sanctuary. Each spring and summer, thousands of gannets and murres nest on narrow ledges above the sea. *Above:* Labrador, Newfoundland's mainland territory, is a vast expanse of bleak, rocky terrain, sparsely populated but rich in mineral resources.

Labrador is a roughly triangular wedge on the eastern coast of mainland Canada. On the west and south it is bordered by the province of Quebec. The Atlantic Ocean is on the southeast; on the northeast is the Labrador Sea, which lies between Labrador and the Danish-owned island of Greenland. Newfoundland island is situated at the mouth of the Gulf of St. Lawrence, 10 to 20 miles (16 to 32 kilometers) from Labrador across the Strait of Belle Isle. The southwestern tip of the island is separated from the province of Nova Scotia by the 68-mile-wide (109-kilometer-wide) Cabot Strait.

As the easternmost province in Canada, Newfoundland is closer to Europe than to many points in North America. For example, the capital city of St. John's is closer to Ireland than it is to the city of Winnipeg in central Canada. Except for the eastern edge of Greenland, Newfoundland is the easternmost part of North America. Because it is so far east, Newfoundland has its own time zone—30 minutes ahead of the rest of Atlantic Canada.

## Rockbound Landscapes

Newfoundland and Labrador are beautiful, but theirs is a stern, uncompromising beauty. The French navigator Jacques Cartier, one of the first Europeans to explore the region, described the coast of Labrador as "stones and frightful rocks and uneven places," and said, "On this entire coast I saw not one cartload of earth, though I landed in many places." On both the island and the mainland, the terrain is indeed rocky and rather desolate. There are no grand mountain peaks, only endless vistas of blunt crags and bluffs, hills and valleys covered with Arctic spruce and tundra, and thousands of lakes and streams. The province's highest point is in the Torngat Mountains in the far north of Labrador. These jagged mountains, eroded over the centuries by rivers and glaciers into a fringe of winding fjords, reach heights of 5,500 feet (1,667 meters). The highest point on the island of Newfoundland is a 2,672-foot (810-meter) peak called Gros Morne in the Long Range Mountains, near the city of Corner Brook.

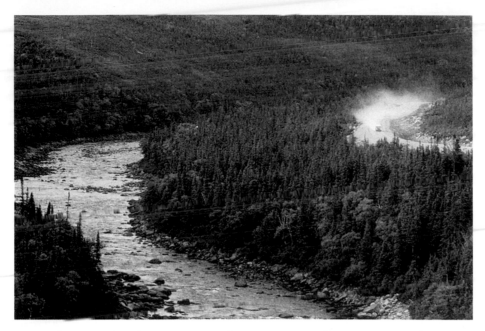

Near Red Bay, Labrador, the Pinware River rushes through a spruce forest. Farther north, the forest gives way to open tundra.

Thousands of years ago, glaciers scraped away most of the soil from Labrador and Newfoundland, leaving the land barren and stony, so much so that Newfoundland has been nicknamed the Rock. But this rocky terrain contains a wealth of mineral resources. Western Labrador has some of the most extensive iron ore deposits in North America.

Although soil suitable for agriculture is scarce in Newfoundland, the province has large forests of evergreen trees, which can grow in shallow, rocky soil. More than 60 percent of Newfoundland island is forested with black spruce, balsam fir, and red and white pine. Labrador, too, has some dense forests of tall evergreens, mostly in the river valleys. But approximately half of Labrador is covered by lichen forests, which consist of slow-growing black spruce, somewhat stunted but hardy enough to survive the region's long winters and short growing seasons, with carpets of lichens and mosses between the trees. The northern part of Labrador is frigid, treeless tundra, where only mosses and occasional dwarf willow and alder shrubs can grow.

The coastlines of both the island and the mainland are greatly indented by many bays and fjords. The island's southeast coast consists of a series of deep bays and coves alternating with

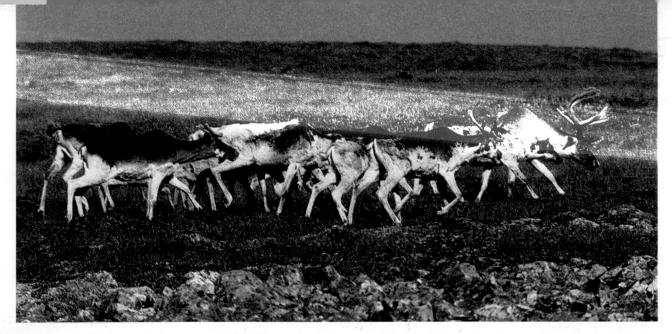

A herd of caribou moves across the grassland of the Avalon Peninsula. Threatened by overhunting during the 19th and early 20th centuries, Newfoundland's two species of caribou have made a comeback in recent decades.

steep headlands and rugged peninsulas. Avalon Peninsula, where the capital is located, is almost an island itself, connected to the rest of Newfoundland by only a narrow neck of land. Fortune Bay, west of Avalon Peninsula, has some of Newfoundland's most dramatic landscapes, with sheer cliffs that rise 590 to 984 feet (180 to 300 meters) from the sea.

## Water and Wildlife

As much as one-fifth of the province of Newfoundland is covered with fresh water. Both island and mainland have thousands of lakes, ponds, streams, and bogs. Many are tiny, but some are quite large and deep. The Smallwood Reservoir in Labrador, for instance, covers approximately 2,500 square miles (6,475 square kilometers) and is the tenth largest freshwater body in Canada.

Newfoundland also has powerful rivers. The Exploits is the longest river on the island, coursing 153 miles (245 kilometers) from Red Indian Lake into Notre Dame Bay on the northeast coast. The Gander is another principal river on the island, with a length of about 109 miles (174 kilometers). Named for the many geese that nest along its shores, the Gander was an important waterway for the island's early European settlers and Natives.

The most powerful of the province's waterways is the Churchill River in Labrador. It runs for 532 turbulent miles (856 kilometers) from Ashuanipi Lake and empties into the Atlantic Ocean near the tiny town of Rigolet, plunging over a 222-foot (75-meter) waterfall on the way. Most of the province's hydroelectric plants are located along the Churchill. Experts believe that the Churchill has the potential to produce more hydroelectric power than any other river in North America.

Newfoundland has another water-related energy resource—peat bogs. Peat is an organic material composed of moss, aquatic grasses, and other plants. In wet, low-lying areas, these plants are periodically covered with water, which causes them to decay, and over time the plant matter is compacted into a dense, spongy substance. When dug out of the bog and dried, peat can be burned like coal to provide heat and energy. Peat is harvested in Newfoundland and elsewhere in Canada, and it is usually cut into bricks or slabs. Once regarded as an old-fashioned or primitive fuel, peat has come to be more highly valued in recent years as an energy resource.

Peat bogs hold more than potential energy. They are also the home of Newfoundland's provincial flower, the pitcher plant. This tube-shaped flower is a meat eater. It produces nectar that attracts insects—the bogs are home to untold millions of mosquitoes and other insects. The hapless victims enter the flower in search of nectar, but the flower is lined with downward pointing bristles from which the insects are unable to escape. They drown in a pool of nectar and water at the bottom of the flower, and the pitcher plant digests them.

Almost 60 species of mammals are native to Newfoundland and Labrador. The province has two species of caribou, woodland and barren ground. The woodland caribou number about 40,000 and live on the island; the barren ground caribou number about 700,000 and live in northern Labrador. For centuries, caribou have been a vital resource for the Native peoples of the region, who hunt them for food and skins. Beginning in the 19th century, however, the caribou were slaughtered in great numbers by white hunters. Since the 1930s,

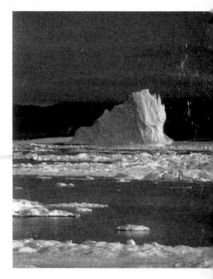

The province's coasts are clogged with pack ice and icebergs during the long, bitter northern winters. In spring, when the ice fields of the northern waters break up, bergs can be seen drifting south past Labrador and Newfoundland.

they have been protected by strict conservation laws. The hunting of caribou, though still permitted, is limited. The caribou population has increased in recent decades, and large herds of these majestic, antlered creatures once again roam across the northern wilderness. Moose, black bear, beaver, lynx, otter, and red fox are also native to the province.

More than 300 species of birds either live in or migrate through Newfoundland. The coastal cliffs and offshore islands are thronged with crowded colonies of seabirds, especially gulls, gannets, and razor-billed auks. Newfoundland is the major breeding center for the Atlantic puffin, a plump black-and-white seabird with a large red-and-gray bill, which has been named the provincial bird. The island's south coast contains what is probably North America's greatest concentration of bald eagles.

Newfoundland is also known for two breeds of dog that originated on the island—Labrador retrievers and Newfoundlands.

Fogs are common, especially in spring and summer. The heavy condensation caused when cold currents from the north meet warmer waters near Newfoundland makes the province one of the foggiest regions in the world.

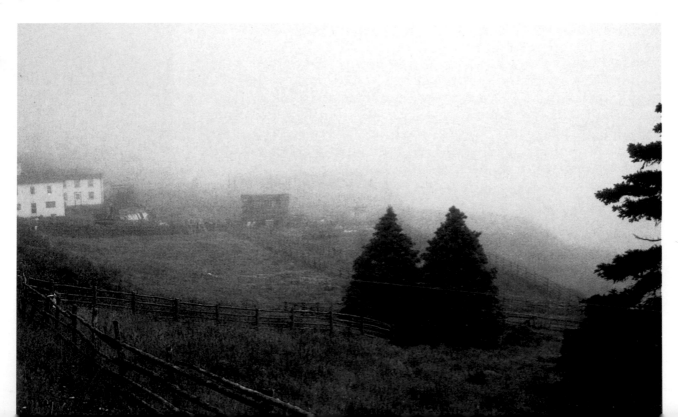

Newfoundlands are large dogs, averaging 28 inches (70 centimeters) in height and 150 pounds (69 kilograms) in weight. Newfs, as they are called, have thick, shaggy coats, usually black but sometimes gray or bronze. They are excellent swimmers and are patient and even-tempered. Newfs have been trained to rescue drowning victims. Labrador retrievers are also large dogs, but they have shorter, sleeker coats. Generally either black or pale yellow, Labs originated as sporting dogs, used by hunters to retrieve fallen birds from water. Like Newfs, they are good swimmers.

## Climate and Weather

Because the province of Newfoundland stretches for nearly 750 miles (1,200 kilometers) from north to south and has both coastal and interior regions, it has a varied climate. The northern and western parts of Labrador are situated in the subarctic zone, where winter temperatures can reach −50 degrees Fahrenheit (−45.6 degrees Celsius). Even midsummer is cool in this region, with July highs reaching 50° or 60°F (10° or 15°C).

Southern and coastal Labrador and Newfoundland island have a milder climate. Winter temperatures in St. John's, the capital, hover around 15° to 25°F (−9° to −4°C). Summer on the island, though brief, is quite lovely. Ocean breezes keep the air crisp and clean, and average high temperatures range from 50° to 60° F (10° to 15°C), although some days are much hotter. Throughout much of the year, the coastal region is shrouded by frequent fogs, which occur when cold air from the interior meets warmer air from the sea.

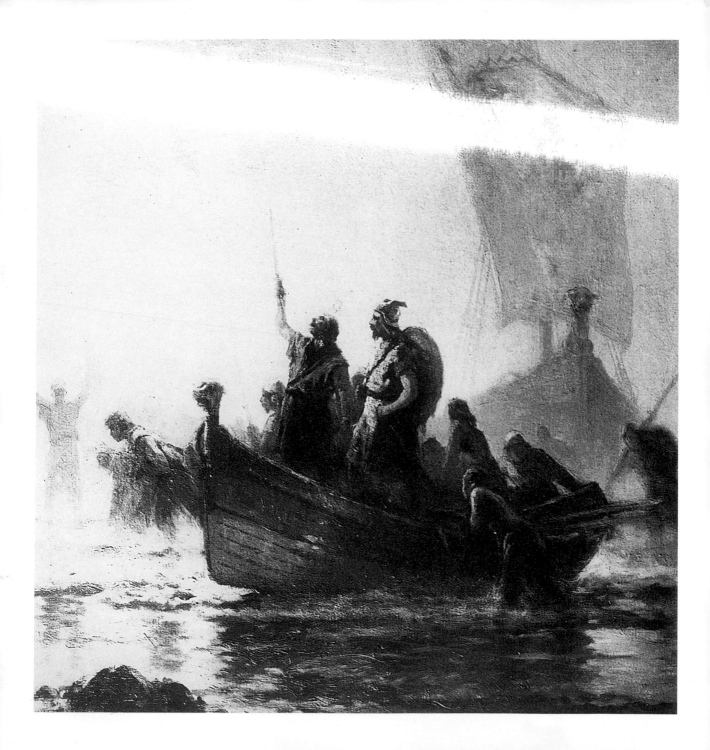

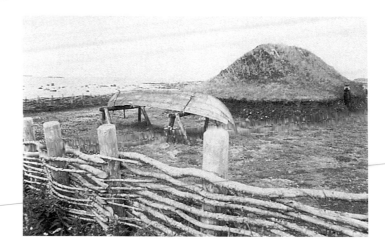

# The History

In 1961, a team of Norwegian archaeologists made one of the most important discoveries in Newfoundland's history: They found the remains of an ancient Viking settlement at l'Anse aux Meadows on the northern peninsula of the island. The findings confirmed that Norse adventurers had found their way across the Atlantic to Newfoundland as early as A.D. 1000. They are now thought to have been the first Europeans ever to see North America.

Norse legends recount that centuries ago certain Vikings sailed from the Norse colonies in Iceland and Greenland to lands farther west. One saga told of Bjarni Herjolfsson, a Viking who was blown off course while sailing from Iceland to Greenland in about A.D. 985. When he finally arrived in Greenland, he spoke of three new lands he had seen in the west. One was forested and hilly, another was forested and flat, and the third was rocky and mountainous. Scholars believe that Herjolfsson had sighted the coasts of Newfoundland, Labrador, and Baffin Island.

Vikings were the first Europeans to visit the shores of Newfoundland. Archaeologists working at L'Anse aux Meadows (above), have uncovered an early Norse settlement that was built around A.D. 1000. The first Viking captain to lead his men ashore in Newfoundland was Leif Eriksson (opposite), the forerunner of European explorers in the New World.

Leif Eriksson was one of the Vikings in Greenland who heard Herjolfsson's story. A dozen years later, Eriksson bought Herjolfsson's ship and went in search of the western lands that Herjolfsson had described. Eriksson and his men landed in three places, which they called Helluland (Rocky Land), Markland (Wooded Land) and Vinland (Wine Land, meaning that it had fruit). Historians now believe that these three landings correspond to the east coast of Labrador, the northern coast of Newfoundland island, and a warm, sheltered bay either on the southern coast of Newfoundland or on Cape Breton Island, Nova Scotia. The Vikings spent the winter in Vinland and returned to Greenland the following spring.

Later, other Norse expeditions visited the new western territory. A few settlements were established in Vinland, including the l'Anse aux Meadows site in Newfoundland, but the settlements were abandoned after attacks by the local Natives, whom the Norse called *skraellings*. The Norse colony in Greenland died out in the 14th century, and knowledge of Vinland and other areas that the Vikings had visited in North America was limited to sagas and legends.

## The Natives

The Vikings did not discover an uninhabited new world. A variety of Native Americans had lived in Labrador and on Newfoundland island for centuries. A tribe who called themselves the Mushuau Innu (Barren Land People) lived in central Labrador and northern Newfoundland. Referred to as the Montagnais-Naskapi by Europeans, these Natives were nomadic hunters of caribou and other mammals. They were adept at traveling across their expansive hunting grounds, using canoes during the summer and snowshoes and toboggans during the winter. When the Europeans came to the region in the 15th and 16th centuries, the Innu helped them to start the fur trade that would eventually spread into most of present-day Canada.

North of the Innu lived the Inuit, who were called Eskimos by the southern tribes. The Inuit lived in small communities scattered

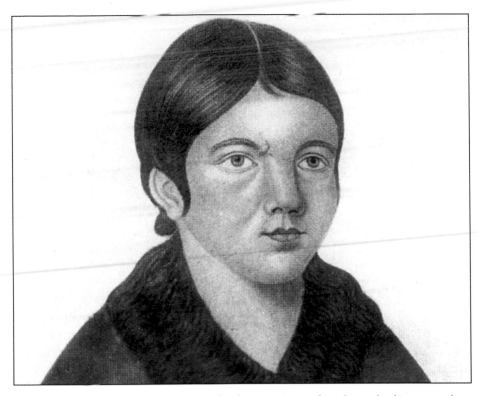

A young woman named Shawnandithet was the last known survivor of the Beothuk, one of the Native peoples of Newfoundland. She died in St. John's in 1829. The Beothuk were wiped out by European aggression, intertribal fighting, and starvation.

throughout the Arctic from Alaska to Greenland, including northern Labrador. They were hunters and gatherers who moved seasonally from one camp to another. They spoke a language known as Inuktitut, which is still spoken by many of the more than 25,000 Inuit who live in Canada today.

The Dorset were another Native people living in Newfoundland at the time of the Viking expeditions. Descended from an ancient Arctic culture, the Dorset lived on Newfoundland island from about 500 B.C. until about A.D. 1500. Distantly related to the Inuit, the Dorset lived in houses built of snow and turf. They hunted sea mammals such as the walrus and the narwhal, an Arctic whale.

The interior and the southern coast of Newfoundland were inhabited by the Mi'kmaq. This Native group lived in villages all along the east coast of North America, from Massachusetts to Quebec. The Mi'kmaq outnumbered the other Native peoples in Newfoundland, and they helped the European settlers survive

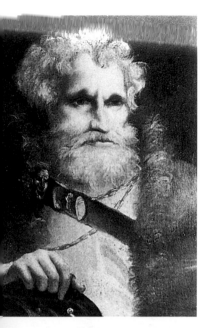

John Cabot, an Italian navigator sailing on behalf of King Henry VII of England, made two voyages to Newfoundland and Labrador in the late 15th century, looking— unsuccessfully—for the fabled Northwest Passage.

their first hard winters in the New World. Several thousand Mi'kmaq still live in Newfoundland; other Mi'kmaq live through out Atlantic Canada.

The Beothuk people lived on the southern and northeastern coasts of the island. They may well have been the first Natives encountered by Europeans in North America; historians now believe that the *skraellings* who fought with the Vikings were either Beothuk or Dorset fishermen. The Beothuk painted their faces with red dye for certain ceremonies, and some scholars have suggested that *redskin,* a term once used for Native Americans, may have referred to this custom. The Beothuk lived in tents covered with bark or animal skin, and they used bows and arrows for hunting and harpoons for fishing. They numbered about 2,000 when English and French settlers began arriving in the 17th and 18th centuries.

The Beothuk were gradually pushed inland by European fishermen who set up camps on the coast, taking over what had once been the Beothuk fishing grounds. In addition, conflicts with the more aggressive Mi'kmaq began to threaten the Beothuk people. Many of them fled the island for the less hospitable shores of Labrador. Sadly, by the early 19th century, the Beothuk people had died out entirely. Some were undoubtedly killed by Europeans and other Natives. Some died of European-introduced diseases, such as tuberculosis and smallpox, against which they had no immunity. Others simply starved to death in the barren regions to which they had been forced to flee. The last surviving Beothuk was a young woman named Shawnandithet, who was captured by English settlers in 1823. Although on the verge of death from starvation, Shawnandithet was able to communicate to her captors an account of the suffering her people had undergone. Her legacy is one of the few clues to the fate of this mysterious people. She died in 1829.

## The European Fishery

During the 14th century, fishermen from Portugal and England made regular visits to the Grand Banks, a rich fishing region not far from Newfoundland. It was generally known that there were islands on the other side of these fishing grounds, but it was not until the end of the 15th century, in 1497, that an official expedition of discovery was launched from Europe. The expedition's captain was John Cabot, an Italian navigator employed by King Henry VII of England to find the hoped-for Northwest Passage, the sea route that was believed to link the North Atlantic Ocean with Asia.

Cabot failed to discover this elusive northern water route to the Orient, because no such route exists south of the Arctic Ocean. But he did land at what is now St. John's, in Newfoundland. In 1501, a Portuguese explorer named Gaspar Côrte-Real made a somewhat more thorough exploration, naming several of Newfoundland's bays and capes. In 1534–35, French explorer

By the end of the 16th century, the seasonal cod-fishing industry was well established in Newfoundland. Fishermen from many nations fished in the island's waters and cured their catch on the shores of its sheltered bays.

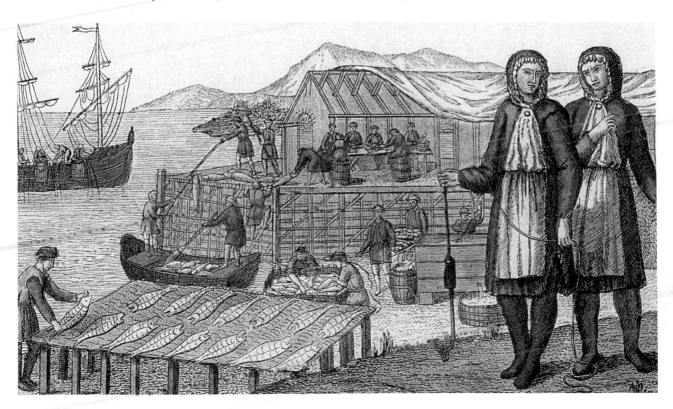

Jacques Cartier sailed through the Cabot Strait and the Strait of Belle Isle, proving that Newfoundland was indeed an island.

By the middle of the 16th century, dozens of fishing boats from England, France, Spain, and Portugal were arriving in Newfoundland waters every summer. The men would haul in huge catches of cod and then set up camps ashore to split, salt, and sun dry the fish. One group of particularly expert fishermen and sailors came from the southeastern corner of Europe's Bay of Biscay, where France and Spain meet. Known as Basques, these hardy seafarers engaged in whaling in the icy waters between Greenland and Canada. Sometime in the 16th century, Basque seamen founded a whaling station at what is now Red Bay, on the southern coast of Labrador. In the 1980s, archaeologists began uncovering the history of this community.

As the end of the 16th century approached, the fragile spirit of cooperation among the fishermen of different nations in Newfoundland's waters began to wear thin. England, greedy for

The Strait of Belle Isle and the coasts of Labrador and Newfoundland were charted in 1766 by Captain James Cook, a British naval officer who later gained fame for his voyages in the Pacific Ocean.

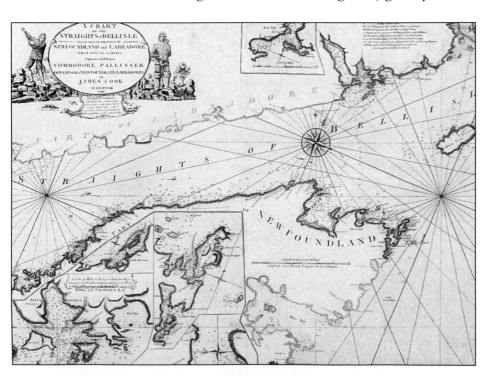

territory and power, sent Sir Humphrey Gilbert to establish a formal claim to Newfoundland. He landed at the port of St. John's on August 3, 1583, and, despite the fact that the harbor was full of ships from Portugal and Spain, he claimed the island for England. The fishermen apparently raised no objection, and Gilbert left a few weeks later. On the way home to England, his ship and crew were lost.

In 1610, King James I of England granted a charter to a group of merchants from the west coast of England. The charter permitted them to establish colonies on the island of Newfoundland, especially on the Avalon Peninsula. The West Country Merchants, as they were called, also received exclusive rights to Newfoundland's offshore fishing grounds.

The merchants' charter caused the development of the Newfoundland colony to lag far behind that of other New World settlements. The West Country Merchants did not want permanent settlers in Newfoundland because such settlers might encroach upon the fishing grounds and compete with their highly profitable seasonal fishing fleets. The merchants went to great lengths to keep settlers out, and they even persuaded the British government to forbid permanent settlement in Newfoundland.

From time to time, however, the Crown did allow communities to be established on the island. The first official colonists, a group of about 40 people, arrived in 1610 with their leader, John Guy. Guy's settlers built a farm, a sawmill, and a stockade in a community they called Cupers Cove (now Cupids Cove) on Conception Bay on the east coast of the Avalon Peninsula. Other settlements followed, but all were threatened by the West Country Merchants.

At the same time, the fishermen had problems of their own: Pirates attacked their boats and looted their stores of fish, supplies, and money. One of the most celebrated pirates in Canadian history was an Englishman named Peter Easton. He led a series of raids against ships from all nations off the coast of Newfoundland, damaging the boats and terrorizing the fishermen.

Starting in 1634, the British government tried to establish law and order in the increasingly rowdy and violent Newfoundland ports. A system called the fishing admiralty was developed.

The captain of the first ship to arrive in a Newfoundland port at the beginning of each summer was named the fishing admiral, or acting governor, for that season. The fishing admiral completely controlled the ships, supplies, and men connected with the fishery. Like the West Country Merchants, the fishing admirals wanted to discourage settlement, and the conflict between the admirals' men and the would-be settlers was bitter and often violent. Houses were burned, and some settlers were beaten or even killed. For a century and a half, the ban on permanent settlement made it very difficult for colonists to clear coastal land for farms and towns. Nevertheless, family holdings and even tiny communities took root in the more remote bays and inlets. Most of these hidden settlements could be reached only by boat. Their inhabitants were called the lost men because they were almost completely cut off from the rest of the world.

## The French and the British

The British were not alone in their desire to control Newfoundland's resources. The Spanish and the Portuguese lost their claims in northern North America by the end of the 16th century, but the French were more tenacious. Newfoundland and the rest of Atlantic Canada became part of a long struggle between France and Britain for control of the New World and for economic supremacy in Europe. By the end of the 17th century, the festering European war had reached the New World, and Newfoundland became a bloody battleground.

For nearly 10 years, battles raged between French and British soldiers and ships. Although the French seemed to have the upper hand in Newfoundland, they fared poorly in Europe and finally conceded defeat. The Treaty of Utrecht, signed in 1713, forced France to give up much of its territory in the New World, including all claims in Newfoundland except for fishing privileges along one stretch of coast. The French Shore, as this region was called, stretched from Cape Bonavista on the east coast around the northern tip of the island and partway down the west coast. Seasonal fishermen from France were the only people allowed on this part

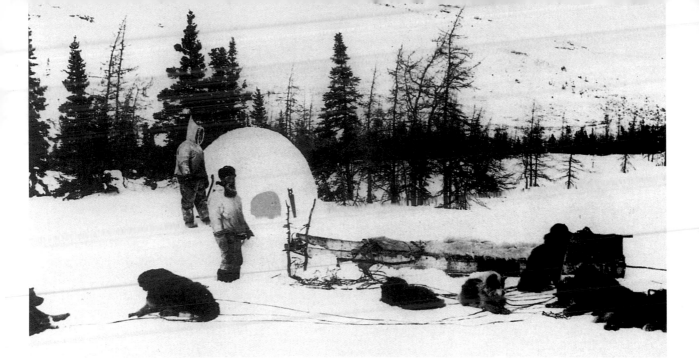

of the island, and no permanent settlement—French or British—took place there until 1904.

However, the Treaty of Utrecht did not end the dispute between the French and the British. Decades later, during the Seven Years' War (1756–63), Newfoundland was once again a bone of contention between the two nations. In 1762, St. John's was lost and then recaptured by the British. The war between the two European powers ended in 1763 with a British victory, and the final battle was fought on Newfoundland soil.

Although the French were soundly defeated, France kept its rights to the French Shore. In addition, Saint Pierre and Miquelon, two small islands south of Newfoundland, were given to the French. They remain part of France today.

## Settlement

A few small settlements were established in Newfoundland during the 18th century. The rate of settlement increased slightly after 1729, when the British crown—disturbed by complaints about the brutality of the fishing admirals—appointed a naval officer as

Northern and central Labrador were almost unknown until the 20th century. This early photograph of a snow hut in the winter landscape near Nain, on the north coast, shows the travelers' dogsled. Sleds are still used in the north, although they have been largely replaced by snowmobiles.

governor of the island. In 1763, at the close of the Seven Years' War, 12,000 people inhabited the island and the southern Labrador shore. After the war, English and Irish colonists arrived to develop and settle the Rock, as Newfoundland soon came to be known. A great wave of immigration occurred during the early part of the 19th century, especially after 1811, when the British government made it legal for colonists to own land and build homes. By 1827, the population had risen to more than 60,000.

As the population increased, so did the demands for better government and local representation. After many months of negotiations with local officials, the British crown granted Newfoundland representative government in 1832. This allowed the colonists to elect an assembly from within their own communities. Most of the real power, however, remained in the hands of a Crown-appointed legislative council. This changed in 1855, when Newfoundland was granted full colonial status, and the power of the elected assembly was greatly increased.

In 1867, some of the other British colonies in North America joined to form a union. This act of confederation resulted in the creation of the Dominion of Canada. The founding members of the Confederation were Canada West (Ontario), Canada East

The St. John's fire of 1892 swept through the tightly packed rows of wooden buildings and left much of the city in blackened ruins. Newfoundlanders at once began rebuilding their capital.

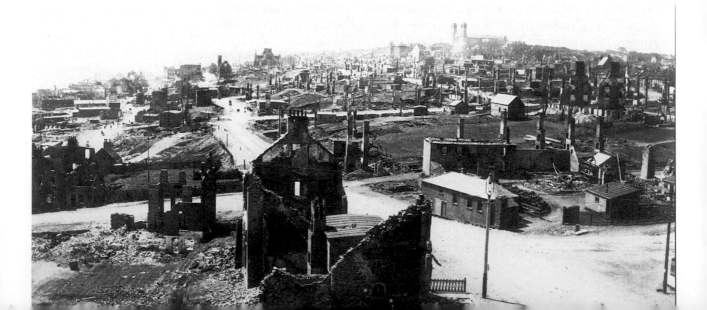

(Quebec), New Brunswick, and Nova Scotia. Newfoundlanders decided against joining the Confederation, because they felt much closer to Great Britain—both geographically and in terms of their national and cultural heritage—than to the rest of Canada. This pro-British spirit endures among many Newfoundlanders today. In addition, the people of Newfoundland could see no compelling economic reasons to join the Confederation. They believed that Newfoundland could rely on its own natural resources and was unlikely to receive much help from the Dominion of Canada.

By the latter part of the 19th century, Newfoundland's salt cod industry was still thriving, pulp-and-paper mills were in operation at Grand Falls, and iron ore mines had opened on Bell Island in Conception Bay. Seal hunters had begun taking huge numbers of fur seals from the ice north of Newfoundland, adding a profitable new industry to the island's economy, while farmers had begun harvesting potatoes. Construction of the island's extensive railway network, begun in 1881, opened up the interior to settlement. By the end of the 19th century, more than 200,000 people lived in the colony of Newfoundland.

## The 20th Century

In spite of its natural resources, Newfoundland was unable to develop a strong and stable economy. Its main industry, the fishery, was particularly vulnerable to changes in the worldwide demand for cod. When this demand declined, as it often did, the value of the colony's fish harvests declined as well. Almost all food had to be imported from Europe or from other parts of North America, often at great cost. Furthermore, the new railroads, mines, and mills were built with borrowed money, and the colony was sinking deeply into debt.

Newfoundland's economy was devastated by World War I (1914–18), which almost completely halted the fishing industry. The colony, however, made a tremendous contribution to the war effort: More than 6,000 of its young men volunteered to fight on the battlefields of Europe. More than 1,000 men from Newfoundland were killed in the war, and almost 2,500 others were wounded.

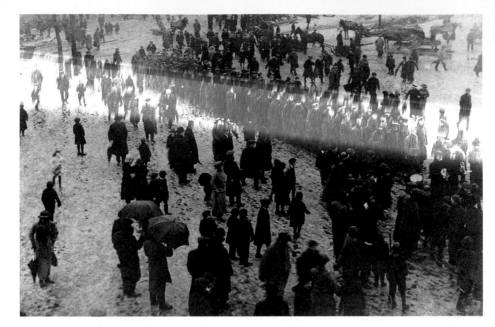

Newfoundland's H Company musters recruits for World War I. In support of Great Britain, the colony sent a great many soldiers, sailors, and airmen to fight in both world wars.

After the war, in recognition of Newfoundland's gallant contribution, Great Britain began to treat Newfoundland as an independent dominion, like Canada or Australia. This status was confirmed by the Statute of Westminster in 1931 and, as a result, Newfoundland actually became an independent country. Unfortunately, independence did not guarantee economic success. The burden of debt caused by the war and the earlier expenses of the railroad construction took a toll on Newfoundland's economy. When the world economy collapsed during the Great Depression of the 1930s, Newfoundland could no longer pay its bills. Turning to Great Britain for assistance, Newfoundland temporarily suspended self-government and became, once again, a British colony in 1934. It was administered by a commission consisting of a governor and six commissioners appointed by the Crown. The commission established programs to improve health care, education, and employment conditions in the colony.

In the meantime, Labrador had been added to the colony. Ownership of the sparsely populated eastern end of the great Labrador-Ungava peninsula had been disputed for many years: The Canadian colony of Quebec claimed the territory, and so did British-controlled Newfoundland. In 1927, a judicial committee in Great Britain ruled that the Labrador coast region did belong to

Newfoundland, under the terms of the 1763 Treaty of Paris. Canada accepted the ruling, and the present boundary between Newfoundland's Labrador territory and Quebec was established.

When World War II(1939–45) broke out in Europe and Asia, Newfoundland was once again ready to make a significant contribution. Thousands of Newfoundlanders served overseas as soldiers, sailors, and airmen, but this time, however, the war also came to Newfoundland. German submarines cruised Newfoundland's waters and torpedoed Bell Island and St. John's, sinking hundreds of ships off the coast. Yet in many ways the war was a boon to the colony. During the war, Newfoundland enjoyed full employment, and its natural resources, including fish, iron ore, and timber, were in great demand. In addition, the United States, Canada, and Britain built several army bases, two large naval bases, and five airports on the island and in Labrador. The money paid to lease these bases was a much-needed boost to the colony's economy. By the end of the war, the administrative commission was able to pay all of Newfoundland's debts and had a surplus of nearly $40 million.

In 1946, the people of Newfoundland faced the task of setting a course for their future. They had three choices: to return to independent dominion status, to remain a British colony administered by the commission, or to join the Canadian Confederation. A referendum was called so that each Newfoundlander could vote on the issue.

One politician who urged the colony to join the Confederation was Joseph R. Smallwood, a dynamic and controversial man who would remain at the forefront of Newfoundland politics for more than two decades. Smallwood wanted Newfoundland to unite with Canada, claiming that "under confederation we would be better off in pocket, in stomach, and in health." Indeed, in the 1940s Canada was a stable, thriving nation that could offer Newfoundland considerable economic support. Funds from Canada's federal government could help build new roads and could sustain families during seasonal slumps in the fishing and forestry industries. And it seemed logical to Smallwood and many other Newfoundlanders that they should become part of the much larger neighboring country that was so willing to offer them assistance.

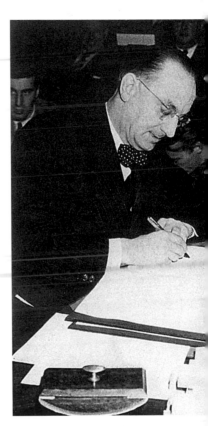

Joseph R. Smallwood signs the document that made Newfoundland part of Canada. After Newfoundland joined the Confederation in 1949, Smallwood became the province's first premier.

On July 22, 1948, the people of Newfoundland voted on the colony's future. By a margin of just four percent, one of Britain's oldest colonies became Canada's newest province. Canada accepted Newfoundland into the Confederation at midnight on March 31, 1949. At the same time, Smallwood became premier of Newfoundland's first provincial government. He held this position until 1972.

Due to an enormous influx of federal money, Newfoundland prospered during the first three decades after Confederation. The fishing industry was modernized, more pulp-and-paper mills were built, and the mineral resources of the island were mined. During the 1950s, the huge iron ore mines of western Labrador came into production as well. But manufacturing, high technology, and financial services—the staples of most modern economies—were severely neglected in Newfoundland.

The economic progress that followed Confederation was to a great extent undermined during the economic recession of the late 1970s and early 1980s. At the beginning of the 1990s, Newfoundland was more dependent than ever on the federal government for support. Overfishing had led to reduced stocks and in 1992 the federal authorities shut down both commercial salmon operations and cod fishing. The province's unemployment rate is high—17 percent—and Newfoundland has the lowest income per person of any province in Canada. Each year, more than 5,000 young people, facing the bleak prospects of building a future in Newfoundland, leave the province to seek work elsewhere.

In addition to its deep-rooted economic problems, Newfoundland is embroiled in two disputes concerning the profits from its natural resources. One of these disputes involves Quebec. Although the courts have awarded Labrador to Newfoundland, Quebec has managed to garner the profits from one of Labrador's most important resources—the hydroelectric power from the Churchill Falls plant. Newfoundland borrowed money from Quebec to build the plant, and in return Newfoundland signed a 40-year agreement to sell the energy produced by the plant to Quebec for a small fraction of its market value. Quebec has been selling electricity to residents of Canada or the United States and reaping huge profits.

Newfoundland has made many attempts to regain control of this valuable resource, by trying to divert water away from the falls and by requesting that the contract be overturned in court. But in 1984 Canada's Supreme Court ruled in Quebec's favor, upholding the contract, and Newfoundland remains at odds with its neighboring province. In 1998, the province signed a cooperative agreement with Quebec to develop an additional 3,200 megawatts of power from the Churchill River project. The deal seeks to lower rates and add millions in revenue.

Newfoundland also disputed Canada's federal government about another potential energy source. The seabed off the coast of Newfoundland contains large reserves of valuable minerals, including oil. One of the largest oil reserves in North America lies in a region under the ocean floor southeast of St. John's. During the 1980s both the federal and provincial governments claimed ownership of the oil fields. Eventually a joint project, the Canada-Newfoundland Offshore Petroleum Board, was established to exploit the resources. In its first year of operation, 1997–98, the Hibernia oilfield produced 20 million barrels of oil.

In spite of its economic misfortunes, Newfoundland possesses a remarkable combination of resources and strengths. Perhaps its greatest asset is its proud and hardy people. Newfoundlanders are sure to meet the challenges of the 21st century with their customary integrity and resolve.

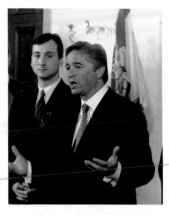

Canadian Premier Brian Tobin of Newfoundland and Labrador, attacks the current level and quality of service provided by Air Canada as he speaks to a news conference on May 8 in Boston.

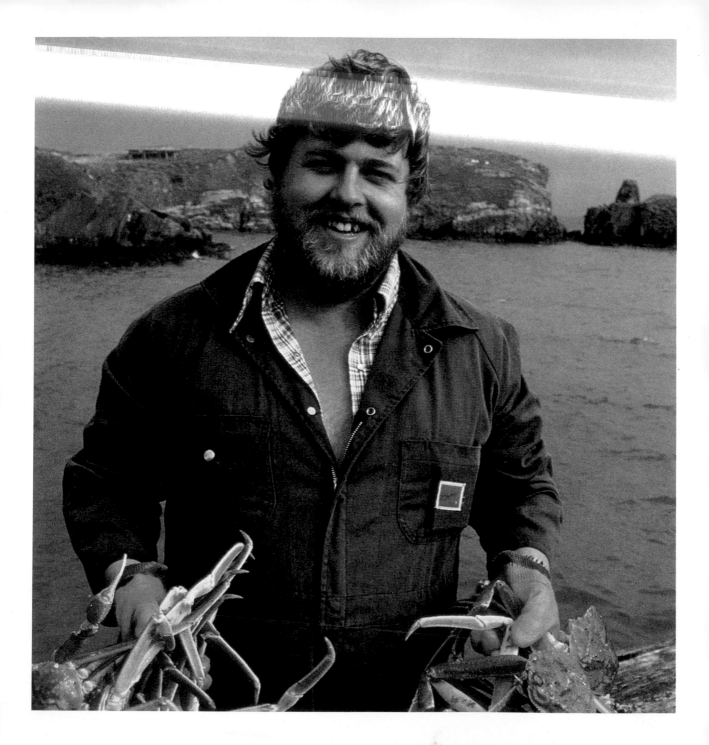

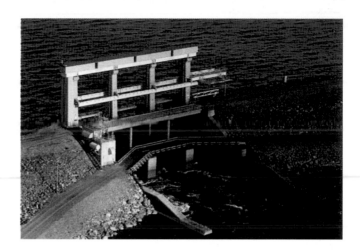

# The Economy

For centuries, Newfoundland has depended on a single major industry, its fishery. In the second half of the 20th century, efforts have been made to develop other industries and businesses to improve the provincial economy.

Like much of the rest of the modern world, Newfoundland has seen the focus of its economy shift from primary industries, such as forestry and fishing, to the financial and service industries. Today more than 70 percent of Newfoundland's workers are employed in financial and service-related occupations such as banking, real estate, health care, tourism, and communications. Tourism in particular is of growing importance, and the province has undertaken a vigorous campaign to attract visitors to the wide open spaces of Newfoundland and Labrador. Nevertheless, resource-based industries remain important.

*Opposite:* A Trinity Bay crabber displays his catch. Fishing was the mainstay of the island for centuries and still plays an important role in the economy.
*Above:* Part of the Churchill Falls hydroelectric plant in Labrador. Energy is one of Newfoundland's most valuable resources, but the province currently receives little of the profit from the electricity produced at this plant.

## The Fishery

Each year, seafood now valued at more than $1 billion is harvested from Newfoundland's waters by about 14,000 fishermen. Most of the catch consists of shellfish. Shrimp, lobster, and snow crab are marketed in the U.S. and United Kingdom and they account for about three-quarters of the money made by fishers. Cod, once the prime fish caught by Newfoundlanders, has been so reduced by over-fishing that only a tiny number are allowed to be harvested each year.

Before the advent of large-scale commercial fishing and fish-processing plants, salted and sun-cured cod were exported in large quantities. Today most of the fish is frozen and processed before being sold.

## Agriculture

With poor soil and an adverse climate, Newfoundland has never had a significant agricultural output. More than 80 percent of the meat, fruit, and vegetables consumed in the province must be imported. Nevertheless, some farming does occur. Many families have small home gardens that help offset the high cost of store-bought produce, and there are some larger commercial farms. Root vegetables are especially well suited to the province's moist, cool climate. Potatoes and turnips are the principal crops, and Newfoundland is

Haymaking on the west coast of the island. Newfoundland has little large-scale agriculture, but there is some good pasturage for livestock; in addition, many people tend small vegetable gardens.

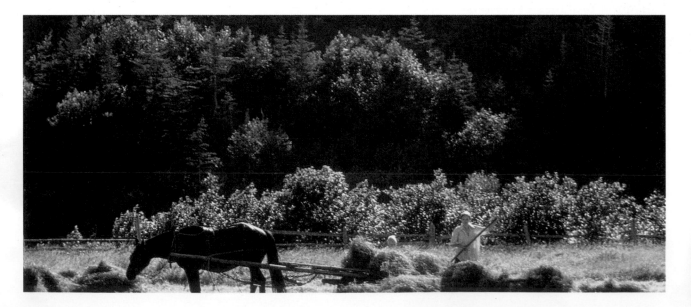

self-sufficient in turnips. Gardeners usually grow cabbage, beets, lettuce, broccoli, and brussels sprouts as well. Blueberries are the major fruit crop. Newfoundland exports more than 2.2 million pounds (1 million kilograms) of this fruit annually. Smaller quantities of strawberries, cranberries, and apples are also grown.

Farmers in Labrador and on the island tend about 4,400 dairy cows, 3,500 beef cattle, and 1,500 calves every year. Newfoundland is totally self-sufficient in egg and poultry production.

One potential agricultural resource is reclaimed peat bogs. New developments in land-use technology have made it possible to drain bogland and plant crops in the mineral-rich soil beneath the water. By 1999, there were 15 vegetable farms established on peatlands (130 hectares) and 14 nursery sod farms (115 hectares). There are also a number of experimental cranberry bogs.

## Forestry

Newfoundland's forests have been harvested for almost as long as its waters have been fished. European visitors in the 16th and 17th centuries used the province's trees for shipbuilding, for fuel, and for timber to build small fishing villages. Today, approximately 40 percent of the island's area consists of productive forestland, and some logging also takes place in Labrador. The forestry trade employs about 10,000 people in lumber mills, logging camps, and pulp-and-paper plants, mostly on the island. Grand Falls, near the center of the island, is the largest forestry center, although Corner Brook on the west coast is gaining importance.

More than 68 percent of the trees felled in the province are made into newsprint, with an annual value of more than $600 million. Unfortunately for the people of Newfoundland, the world market for newsprint is notoriously unstable, and this industry is subject to economic slumps. Often the mills close for months at a time while the workers suffer through bitter periods of unemployment. Another 20 percent or so of Newfoundland's wood is used for fuel. The rest is made into lumber and timber products.

Each year Newfoundland loses a substantial percentage of its potential forest harvest to insects, disease, or forest fires. During the 1970s, the island's forests were severely damaged by an especially lethal infestation of the spruce budworm, an insect that feeds on balsam fir trees. Since then, Newfoundlanders have begun a reforestation program, and they are also trying to develop more efficient and environmentally sound harvesting techniques.

## Mining and Energy

Newfoundland island has most of the province's forestry and agricultural resources, but mainland Labrador leads the way in mineral production. The region holds vast stores of iron, copper, lead, zinc, and other ore. For example, the Voisey's Bay mineral field near Nain, owned by INCO, is estimated to hold hundreds of millions of dollars worth of nickel and cobalt.

Iron is the mainstay of Newfoundland's mining industry, accounting for 90 percent of all mineral products exported from the province. Labrador produces more iron ore than any other area in Canada. In recent years, Newfoundland has mined an average of 20 million tons of iron ore each year. Most of the ore is mined around Labrador City and Wabush in western Labrador.

Other mines throughout Labrador produce smaller quantities of metals and industrial minerals. At one time, copper, zinc, and lead were almost as important to the local economy as iron ore. From the 1920s through the 1960s, the Buchans mine in central Labrador produced some of Canada's highest-grade metals. But after decades of concentrated production, most of the accessible minerals have already been taken from Buchans, and current activity at the mine is limited. Metal ores are not the province's only mining products. Gypsum, silica, and limestone are mined in southwest Labrador.

About 200 miles (320 kilometers) southeast of St. John's, 250 feet (80 meters) under the sea, sits the Hibernia oilfield. It is estimated to hold more than 3 billion barrels of oil, but only about one-third can be recovered using current technology. Other oilfields, including Terra Nova, may hold equal amounts of recoverable oil as well as natural gas. They are expected to begin operations early in the twenty-first century. Many Newfoundlanders

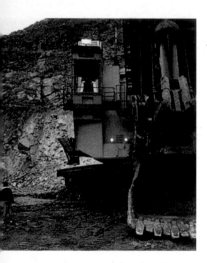

A mine near Labrador City produces hematite, a type of iron ore. Some of Canada's most extensive mineral reserves are located in Labrador; Labrador City and Wabush are the centers of the mining industry.

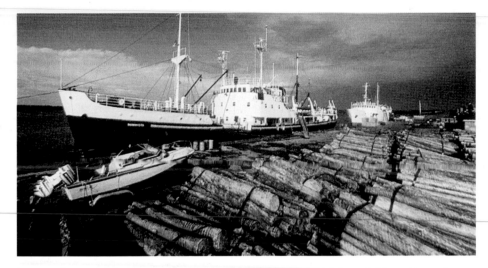

Timber from the province's forests lies stacked on the dock at Goose Bay, southern Labrador's main harbor for both military and commercial shipping.

hope that exploitation of Voisey's Bay minerals and the oil under the sea will soon provide a much needed boost to their economy.

Newfoundland has other energy sources as well. The Churchill Falls hydroelectric power plant is the second largest in Canada and one of the largest in the world. Although most of the power produced at Churchill Falls is exported to Quebec, that plant and others along the Churchill River generate enough electricity to make Labrador self-sufficient in energy production. The technology is not yet in place, however, to transport electricity economically from Labrador to Newfoundland island, so energy is more expensive on the island than on the mainland. A large hydroelectric complex and an oil-burning thermal plant have been built on the island as part of an attempt to increase local energy production.

## Manufacturing

Most manufacturing in Newfoundland involves processing the province's natural resources. The majority of factories are either pulp-and-paper mills or fish-processing plants. Smaller industries that use local materials include boatbuilding yards, lumber mills, and fruit and vegetable canning operations. In addition, small food-processing plants produce staples such as bread, ice cream, soft drinks, and beer. A large phosphorus plant, a paint-manufacturing factory, and a shipbuilding yard rely on imported materials for their operation.

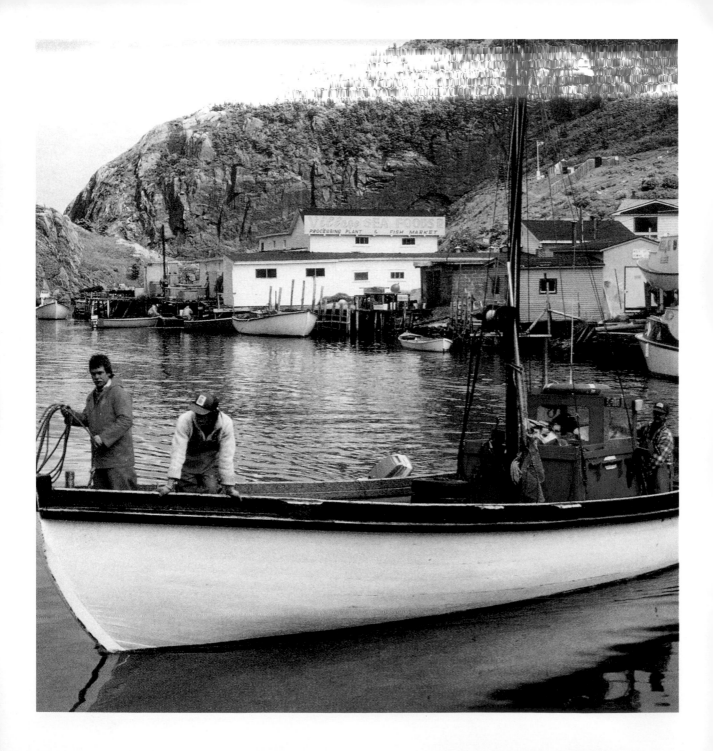

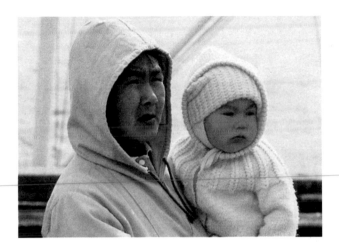

# The People

Life on the Rock, as Newfoundland is fondly known, has never been easy. In the early days of the colony, many settlements were burned to the ground by greedy fishing merchants. Despite these hardships, or perhaps because of them, Newfoundlanders have maintained a hardy and independent spirit. Indeed, they are fiercely loyal to their home, acutely aware of its stark beauty, and respectful of its history and enduring culture.

The people of Newfoundland make up one of the most close knit and ethnically homogenous populations in Canada. (Ethnically homogenous means that a high percentage of the people share the same ethnic background.) The majority of Newfoundlanders are of English or Irish descent, and they have proudly preserved many idioms and traditions from the British Isles.

Visitors to St. John's (pronounced sinJAHNS) and other parts of the Avalon Peninsula will hear a lilting Irish accent. Farther north, the accent is distinctly English, stemming from regions such as Dorset or Devonshire in western England. People throughout

*Opposite:* Fishermen on Quidi Vidi Lake, near St. John's, prepare to tie up. Many Newfoundlanders are as much at home in a boat as on land, the harbor or riverbank remains the center of many communities.
*Above:* An Inuit mother and child. Inhabitants of northern Labrador, the Inuit are related to Arctic peoples across Canada and in Siberia.

the province still use traditional figures of speech, some dating as
far back as 300 years. For example, the word yaffle means an arm-
ful, as in a yaffle of dried fish, and a kinkhorn is an Adam's apple.
Many of these terms died out long ago in England and Ireland, so
English-speaking visitors have a unique opportunity to hear a
centuries-old version of their own language.

Although the English and Irish influences dominate the
province's culture, there are some important minorities. On the
west coast of the island are several small French Canadian fishing
villages. Most of the residents are Acadians, descendants of the
first French settlers in Canada. Another group of French
Newfoundlanders live in western Labrador, near the Quebec
border.

Newfoundland also has an active population of Native peoples, both on the island and in Labrador. In recent years, the Mi'
kmaq people of the island have filed land claims with the federal
and provincial authorities, insisting that European settlers took
land from their tribes illegally. The Mi'kmaq want their tribal ter-
ritories to be returned to them.

Several thousand Inuits and Innus (Montagnais-Naskapis) still
live in Labrador. Most of the Inuit live in the far north, on the
frozen tundra that has been their homeland for centuries. Many of
them continue to follow the traditional Inuit way of life; others
have chosen a more modern course and are involved in the political administration and economic development of northern Canada.
Like the Mi'kmaq, the Inuit have filed land claims against the federal government.

The Innu live in central Labrador. Many Innu are still trying
to maintain their ancestral life-style, hunting caribou in the forests
and fishing in the lakes. But the traditional Innu way of life may be
threatened by a disturbing intrusion. Low-flying military jets from
air bases at Happy Valley—Goose Bay have upset the caribou
herds and other wildlife in the area. The Innu—as well as environ-
mentalists—are concerned that the jets may drive the animals away
or even cause their numbers to diminish. The Innu are negotiating
this and other issues, in particular, control over the Voisey's Bay
nickel deposits, with Canada's federal government.

## Education and Culture

Newfoundland has 600 schools, which accommodate about 140,000 students from kindergarten through 12th grade. The province's first school was established in the 1720s by the Church of England. For centuries, the school system was administered to some extent by the province's various religious denominations. Although the provincial government assumed primary responsibility for the funding of Newfoundland's schools,

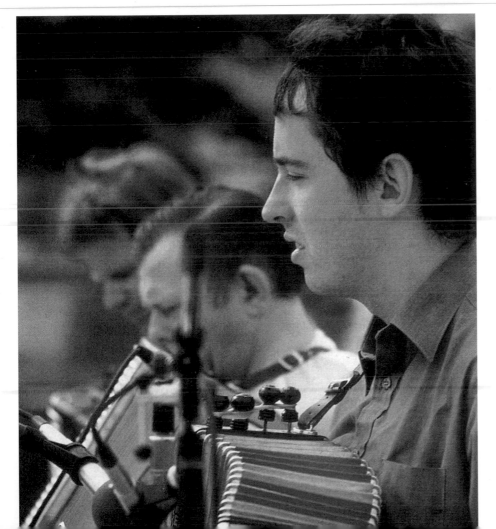

Accordionists perform at the Folk Arts Festival in St. John's. This annual event celebrates the traditional music, dance, and crafts of Newfoundland and Labrador. Because of the province's close-knit communities and geographic isolation, folk songs, stories, and customs have been preserved for centuries.

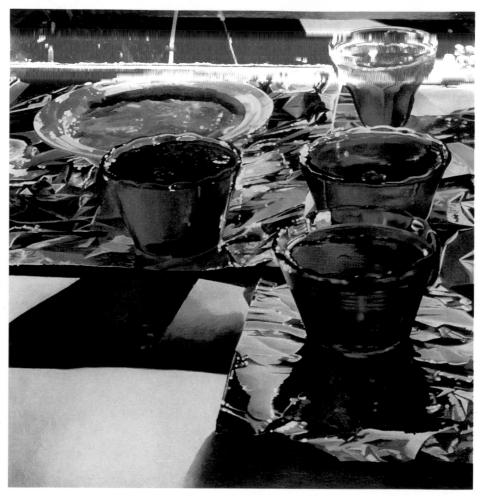

*Red Currant Jelly* (1972) by Newfoundland artist Mary Pratt, hangs in the National Gallery of Canada in Ottawa.

different religious committees assisted the government in making policy decisions and performing administrative functions. However, in September 1997 more than 70 percent of Newfoundlanders voted in favor of creating a secular school system run by the provincial Department of Education and publicly elected school boards.

Newfoundland also has several institutions of higher learning. Vocational schools, many of which focus on marine technology and the fishing industry, can be found in Newfoundland's larger towns. The province's only university is Memorial University, founded in 1925. Located on the northern outskirts of St.

John's, Memorial is the largest and most respected university in Atlantic Canada. Memorial's second campus, Sir Wilfred Grenfell College, is located in Corner Brook. About 12,000 full-time and 4,000 part-time students are enrolled at Memorial. The university offers degrees in arts and sciences, engineering, medicine, and business administration, but regional concerns are its specialty. The Center for Cold Ocean Resources Research, the Marine Sciences Research Laboratory, and the Maritime Studies Research Institute attract marine biologists and engineers from all over North America.

Memorial University also has the province's Folklore and Language Archives, where students learn about the unique folk traditions established and maintained throughout Newfoundland's history. The very nature of the Newfoundland way of life—cultural homogeneity combined with isolation from the rest of the world—enables folkways to stay alive and meaningful in Newfoundland. As a result, the province is a virtual living laboratory for folk historians from around the world.

Many age-old traditions remain a vital part of the province's cultural life today. One particularly colorful activity, performed by both professional actors and the general population, is called mumming. Dressed in costumes, mummers either perform a traditional folk play or parade through the streets in a procession. At Christmastime, mummers of all ages perform the traditional "house visit," in which small groups of costumed and disguised people visit a neighbor's home. Boisterous and full of fun, the mummers try to fool their hosts, who must try to identify their rowdy guests.

Folk music is an important part of Newfoundland culture. Lively Irish jigs and old English folk songs are heard throughout the province. In the 1990s one Newfoundland group called "Great Big Sea" gained popularity throughout Canada for its modern renditions of sea shanties and reels. This Petty Harbour band has won numerous "Entertainer of the Year" honors at the East Coast Music Awards and sold nearly one-half million records in Canada in the last few years.

The age old art of storytelling also remains an integral part of the modern Newfoundland cultural scene. Coffeehouses and taverns are often the sites of local storytelling performances. The annual Newfoundland Drama Festival, which was first held in 1950, showcases both professional and amateur storytellers and playwrights from all over the province.

Newfoundland has produced a number of internationally known writers and painters. E. J. Pratt (1883–1964), recognized as one of Canada's finest poets, wrote poems that present realistic and unsentimental looks at maritime life in his native province. One of his most important works was *Newfoundland Verse* (1923).

David Lloyd Blackwood, born in Wesleyville on Bonavista Bay in 1941, is perhaps Newfoundland's best-known visual artist; he is both a printmaker and painter. Blackwood's work reflects the province's unique maritime history, particularly the sea captains of Bonavista Bay. Considered one of Canada's most important etchers, Blackwood now lives in Toronto.

Throughout the province, museums and historical societies have collected impressive displays of irreplaceable artifacts that tell the story of Newfoundland and its people. The Newfoundland Museum in St. John's, for instance, has some of the few relics left by the extinct native Beothuk culture. At L'Anse aux Meadows, a museum depicts the way of life of the ancient Vikings who were the first Europeans to see North America.

## Sports and Recreation

The sporting tradition in Newfoundland goes back to the early 19th century. The oldest organized sporting event in North America is St. John's Regatta Day, which has taken place on Quidi Vidi Lake near the capital on the first Wednesday of every August since 1826. Oarsmen from across the province compete in a 2.5-mile (4-kilometer) race in traditional 6-oared craft. The daylong regatta attracts 50,000 people each year.

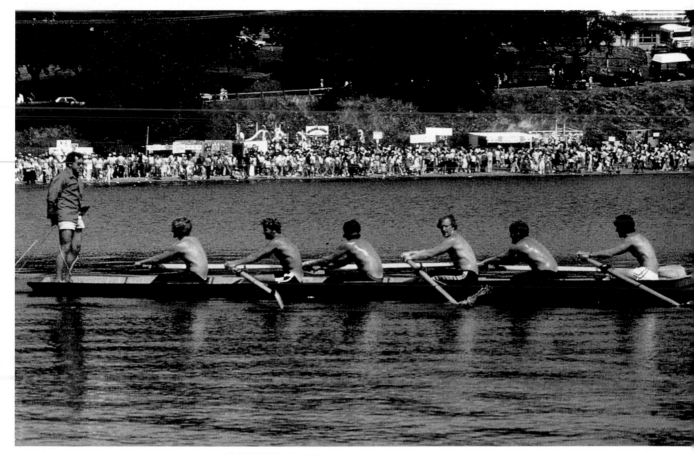

Newfoundlanders enjoy a variety of outdoor activities, which also attract tourists who want an active, nature-oriented vacation. Bird-watchers, backpackers, and campers find plenty to do in Newfoundland and Labrador. Sports fishermen flock to the province's lakes and rivers as well as to its seacoasts. Hunters can obtain permits for game on both the island and the mainland. Winter brings ski season. Labrador has some of the best cross-country trails on the east coast of North America, and the Marble Mountain ski resort near Corner Brook on the island is known for its abundant snow and excellent downhill ski trails.

St. John's Regatta Day, a rowing contest, is the oldest sporting event in North America. It has been held since 1826.

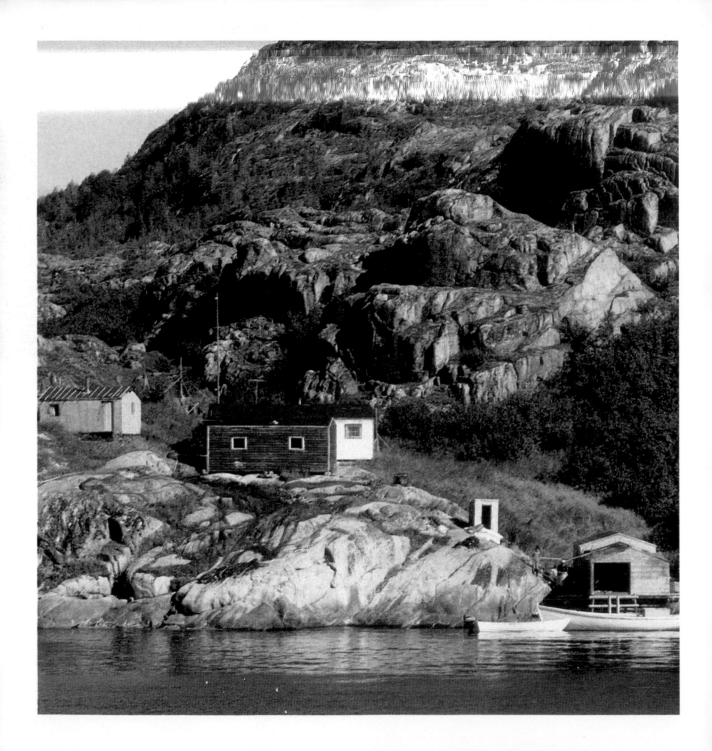

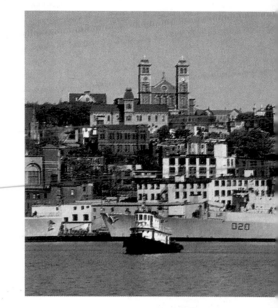

# The Communities

More than 60 percent of all Newfoundlanders live in towns, mostly in St. John's or other communities on the Avalon Peninsula. A few towns have sprung up in the interiors of both the island and the mainland. Many Newfoundlanders, however, still inhabit the small communities called outports that were founded as the region was originally explored and settled. Outports dot the fringes of both the island and the mainland. Some are as large as towns or villages, others are just a huddle of buildings where a few families live, but all are situated on the coast.

Many outports cannot be reached by road and are accessible only by boat or ship. Set in sheltered inlets to protect them from the harsh Atlantic climate, most Newfoundland outports have at least one church, a school, a store, and a post office. One essential feature of the local landscape is the docks, where fishing boats, small motor launches, and weather-worn rowboats may be seen. The fishery provides the livelihood for most of the outport residents, and fish-processing plants are located close to many of these communities. After Newfoundland became part of Canada

*Opposite:* A Labrador outport. The coasts of the island and the mainland are dotted with these tiny settlements, many of which can be reached only by boat.
*Above:* The harbor at St. John's, the province's capital.

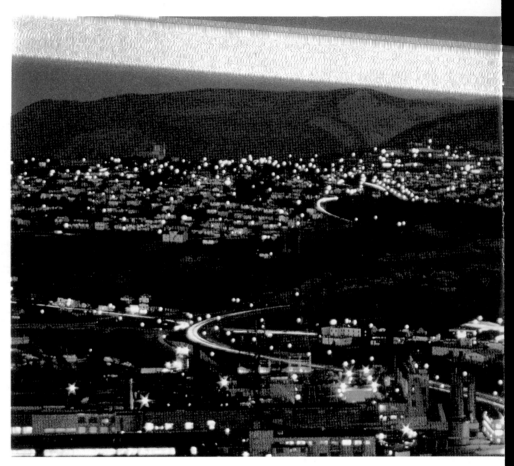

Corner Brook, on the west coast of the island, is the province's second largest city.

in 1949, government agencies succeeded in closing some of the outports and moving families into the newer towns, where social services and jobs were more readily available. Nevertheless, more than 1,000 outports have survived.

The stark beauty of Newfoundland's cities, towns, and outports is offset by the whimsical charm of their names. Place names such as Come by Chance, Ha Ha Bay, Black Tickle, Heart's Content, Joe Batt's Arm, Witless Bay, and Flower's Cove commemorate episodes in local history, or reflect the relief experienced by early mariners or settlers at having found a safe haven after the rough Atlantic crossing.

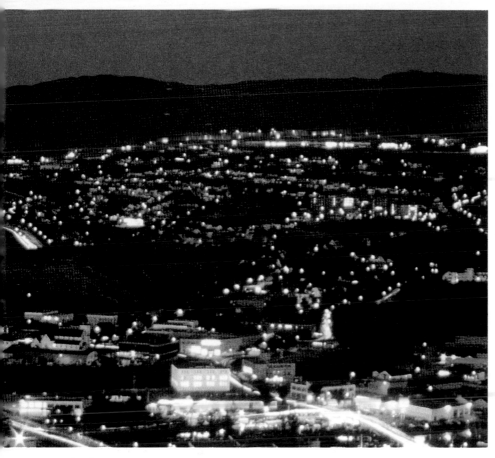

## St. John's

According to legend, in 1497, on the Roman Catholic holiday called the Feast of St. John the Baptist, explorer John Cabot sailed into the entrance of a snug, protected harbor on the southeast corner of the "new found land" and named the port St. John's in honor of the saint. Fishermen began to use the sheltered bay, and it was not long before a settlement had taken root there. Some historians believe St. John's to be the oldest European settlement in the New World north of Mexico. Today it is both the capital and principal city of the province.

Like Newfoundland itself, St. John's has always looked to the sea for its livelihood. Throughout much of its early history, it was one of the most important ports in eastern Canada. English, French, Basque, and Portuguese fishermen made its magnificent, almost landlocked harbor their haven from the rough and unpredictable Atlantic Ocean. More recently, however, the harbor at St. John's has been overshadowed by other eastern ports, especially Halifax, Nova Scotia. Most goods that come to Newfoundland island from the mainland now arrive by truck, ferried from Nova Scotia to Port aux Basques at the southwestern tip of the island. Nevertheless, the sea remains an integral part of the cityscape.

St. John's is built upon a series of steep hills, which protect the harbor below from high winds and bad weather. The sea is visible from almost every vantage point, especially in the oldest part of the city, where narrow, brightly painted wooden houses line the steep streets. Unfortunately, not much remains of old St. John's because the city was almost completely destroyed by fire several times in the 19th century. The most recent large fire, which left 13,000 people homeless, occurred in 1892. After each fire, the city was painstakingly rebuilt.

Signal Hill, a mass of granite near the mouth of the harbor, offers one of the best views of the city and the harbor. The hill is a natural fortress that has played a significant role in the defense of Newfoundland over the centuries. Every summer, historic battles are reenacted there during a monthlong pageant. At the top of Signal Hill stands Cabot Tower. Built in 1897 to commemorate the 400th anniversary of the discovery of Newfoundland by John Cabot, the tower was the site of an important 20th-century event: the reception of the first transAtlantic radio message in 1901 by Italian inventor Guglielmo Marconi.

More than 101,000 people live in St. John's, most of them employed by the federal, provincial, and municipal government agencies that have headquarters in this surprisingly cosmopolitan city. St. John's is also the center of artistic activity in Newfoundland. The Newfoundland Symphony Orchestra is based there, and a number of theater groups have called the centre home, including CODCO, a repertory company that specializes in character comedy.

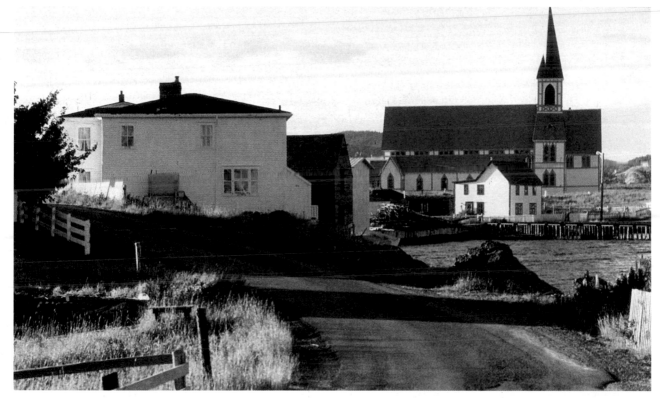

CODCO's half-hour comedy show was televised on the Canadian Broadcasting Corporation (CBC) in the 1990s and several of its performers have gone on to star in the satirical television program "This Hour Has 22 Minutes." Memorial University's Arts and Culture Centre presents performances of Shakespearean plays and other productions. Restaurants, department stores, and nightclubs share the cityscape with parks, office towers, and quaint, old houses. Water Street, thought to be the oldest street in North America, is the center of the shopping district.

Trinity, a seaside hamlet on the island's north coast. Many Newfoundlanders live in small communities such as Trinity, but each year thousands of young people move to the cities or to other provinces in search of better job opportunities.

## Corner Brook

Corner Brook, the second largest city in Newfoundland, is located on the opposite side of the island from St. John's. Corner Brook is often called the province's western capital. It is an industrial city of almost 22,000 inhabitants that was formed in 1956 when 4 towns—Curling, Corner Brook West, Corner Brook East, and Townsite—merged.

The forestry trade has been at the center of Corner Brook's growth and development since 1864, when a sawmill opened in the area. In 1923, the Newfoundland Power and Paper Company was formed, and the modern city developed around this large group of resource-related companies. A power plant, located in nearby Deer Lake, has helped to fuel the city's continued economic growth.

In general, the west coast is colder in the winter and warmer in the summer than the east coast. Corner Brook receives more than 150 inches (381 centimeters) of snow every year. This dependable snowfall has led to the development of some excellent ski areas in the Corner Brook region.

## Labrador

The mainland portion of Newfoundland is a sparsely populated wilderness speckled with a few industrial towns. Fewer than 30,000 people live in Labrador. Its population may be small, but Labrador has an abundance of natural resources that have made it one of the most hotly contested regions of Canada. Quebec and Newfoundland have been in dispute over the ownership of Labrador for centuries. At present, Newfoundland has the upper hand: The Constitution Act of 1982 confirmed that Labrador was indeed part of Newfoundland.

Labrador's extended seacoast, indented by innumerable fjords, bays, and inlets, has attracted fishermen for nearly a thousand years. Today several ports on the barren, rocky coast provide seasonal docks for ships from Canada, Europe, Japan, and Russia. But relatively few people are willing to brave the stark winters of Labrador's coastal regions. Red Bay, located on the south coast where the climate is most temperate, has only 275 residents.

The interior of Labrador is far more populous than the coast. At the center of the region is Happy Valley—Goose Bay, a town of about 8,655 people formed when the separate communities of Happy Valley and Goose Bay amalgamated in 1974. During World War II, Goose Bay was the site of the world's largest military airport. Used by the Royal Canadian Air Force, the United States Air Force, and the Canadian Army, the airport employed more than 3,000 Labradorians. The base is currently a refueling and support installation for the air forces of many nations. Surrounded by some of the most beautiful fishing and hunting grounds in North America, Happy Valley—Goose Bay is also the center of Labrador's tourism industry during summer and autumn

Labrador City, an industrial center, and the smaller community of Wabush are located west of Happy Valley—Goose Bay, near the Quebec border. Slightly more than 8,400 people live in Labrador City, making it the largest town on mainland Newfoundland. Most local workers are employed by one of the many iron ore mining plants that have been founded since ore was discovered there in 1892. Labrador City experienced a population boom after 1961, when the Labrador peninsula was linked by railroad with Quebec.

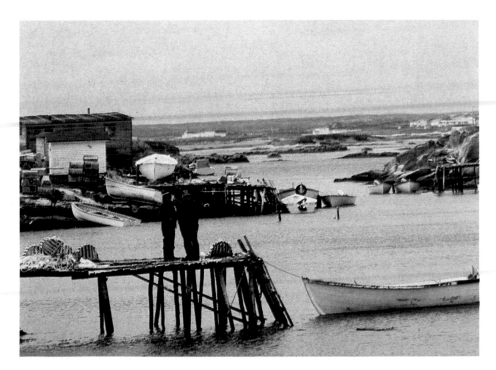

For centuries, Newfoundlanders wrested their living from the sea. Although fishing is no longer central to the province's economy, life still revolves around the sea. Boats are as familiar as cars to many Newfoundlanders.

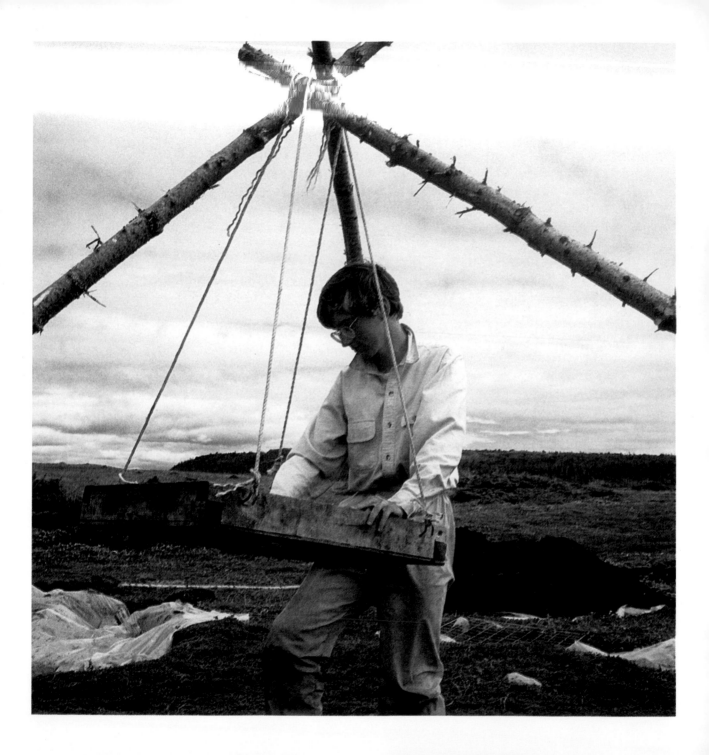

# Things to Do and See

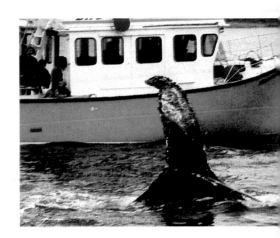

- **Signal Hill National Historic Park and Cabot Tower,** St. John's: Set atop a rocky headland, this park commemorates a number of important events in Newfoundland history, including the arrival of explorer John Cabot in 1497 and the first transatlantic radio transmission in 1901. Breathtaking views of St. John's and the harbor may be enjoyed from Cabot Tower. An interpretive center displays artifacts documenting the city's history.

- **Cape Spear,** 10 miles (16 kilometers) south of St. John's: This is North America's closest point to Europe and the site of one of Canada's oldest surviving lighthouses, built in 1836.

- **L'Anse aux Meadows:** This UNESCO World Heritage Site is a recreation of the sod village and living quarters built and inhabited by the Vikings in the 10th century A.D.

- **Arts and Culture Centre,** St. John's: The site of the city's main theater, which seats 1,000. The Arts and Culture Centre also includes a large lending library, an art gallery, and several rehearsal rooms.

*Opposite:* An archaeologist at Port au Choix on Newfoundland's west coast is helping to excavate a several-thousand-year-old settlement of the Dorset, one of Newfoundland's Native peoples. *Above:* Once hunted to near extinction, whales now make a different kind of contribution to the provincial economy: They inspire scores of whale-watching tours each year.

- The Newfoundland Museum, St. John's: Displays relics of the region's early inhabitants and cultural settlements, including those of the extinct Beothuk people and the Basque whalers. The museum also has artifacts from many of the vessels that have been shipwrecked on Newfoundland's shores.

- **Gander Airport Aviation Exhibition,** Gander: Newfoundland's important role in pioneer aviation, both transatlantic and domestic, is recounted in documents and displays in this small museum located in an airport terminal building.

- **Gros Morne National Park,** 75 miles (120 kilometers) north of Corner Brook: Covering 750 square miles (1,942 square kilometers) of seacoast and mountains, this park has been designated a UNESCO World Heritage Site. It contains sites where archaeologists have uncovered relics of Dorset, Inuit, and Beothok habitations. It also has rugged hiking trails, facilities for swimming and boating (and surprisingly warm water during the summer), and cross-country ski trails.

- **Terra Nova National Park,** 145 miles (232 kilometers) northwest of St. John's: Canada's easternmost national park, Terra Nova is a naturalist's paradise. The park's starkly beautiful landscape features six lakes carved out by glaciers thousands of years ago. Careful observers may see whales and seals off the shore. Numerous seabirds nest in the region, and animals of many species roam the park.

- **Marble Mountain Ski Resort,** near Corner Brook: Ski runs extend for more than a mile (a kilometer and a half), and drops of about 700 feet (213 meters) make this one of the best ski resorts in Newfoundland.

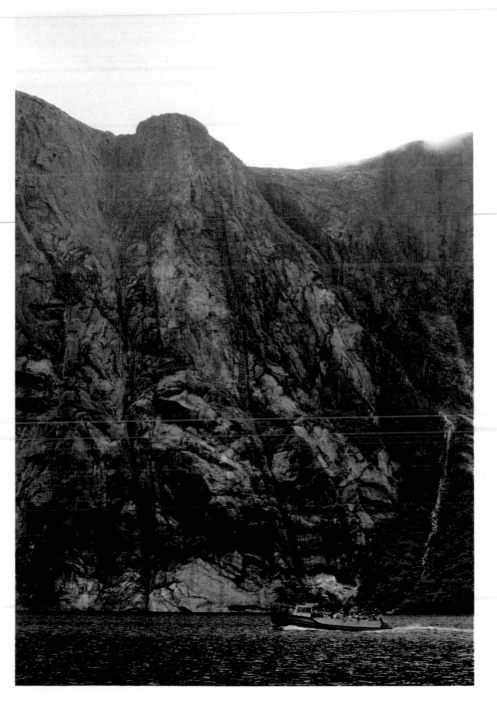

Tourists in a charter boat cruise past billion-year-old cliffs in Gros Morne National Park.

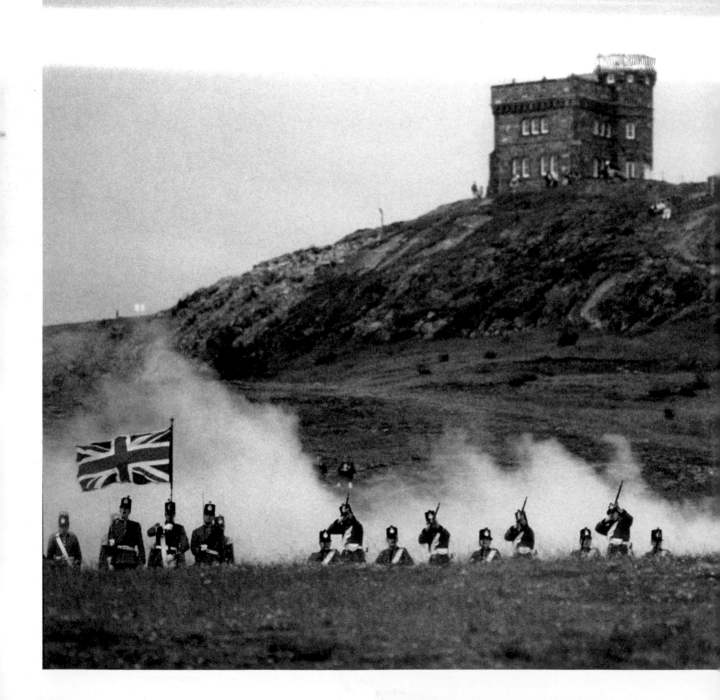

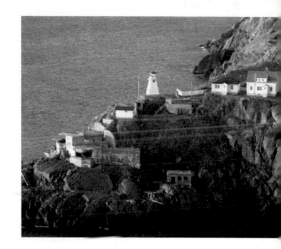

# Festivals & Holidays

*Kelligrew's Soiree,* Conception Bay: Made famous by folksinger Johnny Burke, this annual festival of eating and merriment is held in July and includes a regatta for the neighboring towns.

*Regatta Day,* St. John's: Held on the first Wednesday of every August, or "the first fine day thereafter," this is the oldest sporting event in North America. Teams of rowers in racing shells compete on Quidi Vidi Lake. A fair, parade, and festival entertain the more than 50,000 people who attend this annual event.

*Newfoundland and Labrador Folk Festival,* St. John's: Folksingers and musicians from all over Canada, the United States, and Europe flock to St. John's during August for this international musical celebration of folk traditions.

*Winter Carnival,* throughout the province: Corner Brook, Mount Pearl, and Labrador City are just few of the Newfoundland communities that host winter carnivals. From January to March, parades, snow-sculpture contests, skiing and skating parties, and other events help to make the province's long winter more enjoyable.

*Newfoundland and Labrador Drama Festival,* St. John's: Held in mid-April, this event features theater, storytelling, and dance presentations.

*Opposite:* Each year, battles between the English and the French are reenacted at Signal Hill in St. John's. Cabot Tower, atop the hill, is where Marconi received the first transatlantic radio message. *Above:* The Battery, near St. John's, was built by the British army as a coastal defense post during the American War of Independence. During the War of 1812, it protected the colony from a possible U.S. invasion. Today it is a popular—and picturesque—tourist attraction.

# Chronology

| | |
|---|---|
| 1000 | Vikings build a settlement at L'Anse aux Meadows. |
| 1497 | John Cabot sails into the harbor at St. John's. |
| 1610 | The West Country Merchants receive control of the Newfoundland fishery. |
| 1713 | The Treaty of Utrecht recognizes British sovereignty over Newfoundland. |
| 1811 | The British government allows settlement in Newfoundland. |
| 1832 | The Newfoundland settlers are permitted to elect an assembly. |
| 1855 | Newfoundland is given full colonial status. |
| 1867 | Newfoundland decides not to join the new Canadian Confederation. |
| 1892 | St. John's is devastated by a huge fire. |
| 1927 | Mainland Labrador is awarded to Newfoundland. |
| 1931 | The British government recognizes Newfoundland as an independent dominion. |
| 1934 | Newfoundland waives its dominion status, becoming a colony once again, and a British-appointed commission takes over its administration. |
| 1949 | Newfoundland becomes part of Canada. Joseph R. Smallwood becomes the province's first premier. |
| 1984 | The Supreme Court of Canada rules that offshore oil belongs primarily to the federal government. |
| 1989 | Newfoundland celebrates its 40th year as a Canadian province. |
| 1997 | 500th Anniversary Celebration of Cabot's arrival |
| 1998 | A cooperative agrecment with Quebec to develop an additional 3,200 megawatts of hydro-electricity from the Churchill River power system seeks to lower utility rates and add millions in revenue. |
| 1999 | Newfoundland hosts the Canada Winter Games. |

# Further Reading

Armitage, Peter: *The Innu*. New York: Chelsea House, 1991.

Boudreau, Amy. *Story of the Acadians*. Gretna, LA: Pelican, 1971.

Davidson, James W., and Joan Rugge. *Great Heart: The History of a Labrador Adventure*. New York: Viking Penguin, 1988.

Fingard, Judith. *Jack in Port: Sailortowns of Eastern Canada*. Toronto: University of Toronto Press, 1982.

Frideres, James. *Canada's Indians: Contemporary Conflicts*. Englewood Cliffs, NJ: Prentice-Hall, 1974.

Haaland, Lynn. *Acadia Seacoast: A Guidebook for Appreciation*. Edited by Louise Mills and Mercy Johnson. Manset, ME: Oceanus, 1984.

Hocking, Anthony. *Newfoundland*. Toronto and New York: McGraw-Hill Ryerson, 1978.

Holbrook, Sabra. *Canada's Kids*. New York: Atheneum, 1983.

Horwood, Harold A. *Newfoundland*. New York: St. Martin's Press, 1969.

Ingstad, Anne Stine. *The Norse Discovery of America*. Oslo, Norway: University of Oslo Press, 1985.

Law, Kevin. *Canada*. New York: Chelsea House, 1999.

Marshall, Ingeborg. *The Boethuk of Newfoundland: A Vanished People*. St. John, Newfoundland: Breakwater Books Ltd., 1999.

McNaught, Kenneth. *The Penguin History of Canada*. New York: Penguin Books, 1988.

Mowat, Farley. *The Rock Within the Sea: A Heritage Lost*. Boston: Little, Brown, 1969.

Neary, Peter, and Patrick O'Flaherty. *By Great Waters: A Newfoundland and Labrador Anthology*. Toronto: University of Toronto Press, 1974.

Wallis, Wilson Dallam. *The Micmac Indians of Eastern Canada*. Minneapolis: University of Minnesota Press, 1955.

Whiteley, George. *Northern Sea, Hardy Sailors*. New York: Norton, 1982.

Woodcock, George. *The Canadians*. Cambridge: Harvard University Press, 1980.

# Index

ACKNOWLEDGMENTS
The Bettmann Archive: p. 20; Diana Blume: p. 6; Canadian Parks Service/
J. Steeves: p. 5, Churchill Falls (Labrador) Corporation: p. 33; Homer Green: pp.
8, 12, 14, 38, 46, 55; Gros Morne National Park, Canadian Parks Service: p. 57;
Industry, Science and Technology Canada photo: pp. 13, 32, 34, 37, 39, 41, 53,
59; Library of Congress: p. 16; National Archives of Canada: pp. 19 (C38862),
21 (C70648), 22 (NMC-1722); National Gallery of Canada, Ottawa: p. 42;
Keith Nicol, Cornerbrook, Newfoundland: cover, pp. 3, 11, 17, 47, 48–49; Not-
man Photo Archives, McCord Museum of Canadian History: p. 25; Courtesy of
Provincial Archives of Newfoundland and Labrador: pp. 26 (NA1578), 28 (B3-
174), 29 (B16-155); Reuters/ Bettmann Archive: p. 31; Joe Roman: pp. 36, 54;
Debora Smith: p. 7; Wayne Sturge, Department of Development, Government of
Newfoundland and Labrador: p. 45; Michel Thérien: pp. 9, 58; Courtesy of
Tourism Canada, Ottawa: p. 51.

Suzanne LeVert has contributed several volumes to Chelsea House's CANADA IN THE 21ST CENTURY series. She is the author of four previous books for young readers. One of these, *The Sakharov File*, a biography of noted Russian physicist Andrei Sakharov, was selected as a Notable Book by the National Council for the Social Studies. Her other books include *AIDS: In Search of a Killer*, *The Doubleday Book of Famous Americans*, and *New York*. Ms. LeVert also has extensive experience as an editor, first in children's books at Simon & Schuster, then as associate editor at *Trialogue*, the magazine of the Trilateral Commission, and as senior editor at Save the Children, the international relief and development organization. She lives in Cambridge, Massachusetts.

**George Sheppard,** General Editor, is an instructor at Upper Canada College in Toronto. Dr. Sheppard earned his Ph.D. in Canadian History at McMaster University in Hamilton, Ontario and has taught at McMaster, Laurentian, and Nipissing Universities. His research specialty is Canadian Social History and he has published items in *Histoire sociale/Social History*, *The Canadian Historical Review*, *The Beaver*, *Canadian Social Studies*, *The Annual Bulletin of Historical Literature*, *Canadian Military History*, *The Historical Dictionary of the British Empire*, *The Encyclopedia of POW's and the Internment*, and *The Dictionary of Canadian Biography*. He has also worked as a historical consultant for educational material in both multimedia and print format and has published a book entitled *Plunder, Profit and Paroles: A Social History of the War of 1812 in Upper Canada*. Dr. Sheppard is a native of Timmins, Ontario.

**Pierre Berton,** Senior Consulting Editor, is the author of 34 books, including *The Mysterious North*, *Klondike*, *Great Canadians*, *The Last Spike*, *The Great Railway Illustrated*, *Hollywood's Canada*, *My Country: The Remarkable Past*, *The Wild Frontier*, *The Invasion of Canada*, *Why We Act Like Canadians*, *The Klondike Quest*, and *The Arctic Grail*. He has won three Governor General's Awards for creative nonfiction, two National Newspaper Awards, and two ACTRA "Nellies" for broadcasting. He is a Companion of the Order of Canada, a member of the Canadian News Hall of Fame, and holds 12 honorary degrees. Raised in the Yukon, Mr. Berton began his newspaper career in Vancouver. He then became managing editor of *McLean's*, Canada's largest magazine, and subsequently worked for the Canadian Broadcasting Network and the *Toronto Star*. He lives in Kleinburg, Ontario.